Advances in Mobile Health Technology

The COVID-19 pandemic upended the lives of many and taught us the critical importance of taking care of one's health and wellness. Technological advances, coupled with advances in healthcare, has enabled the widespread growth of a new area called *mobile health* or *mHealth* that has completely revolutionized how people envision healthcare today. Just as smartphones and tablet computers are rapidly becoming the dominant consumer computer platforms, mHealth technology is emerging as an integral part of consumer health and wellness management regimes.

The aim of this book is to inform readers about the this relatively modern technology, from its history and evolution to the current state-of-the-art research developments and the underlying challenges related to privacy and security issues. The book's intended audience includes individuals interested in learning about mHealth and its contemporary applications, from students to researchers and practitioners working in this field.

Both undergraduate and graduate students enrolled in college-level healthcare courses will find this book to be an especially useful companion and will be able to discover and explore novel research directions that will further enrich the field.

Chapman & Hall/CRC Healthcare Informatics Series

Process Modeling and Management for Healthcare
Carlo Combi, Giuseppe Pozzi, Pierangelo Veltri

Consumer Health Informatics
Enabling Digital Health for Everyone
Catherine Arnott Smith, Alla Keselman

Statistics and Machine Learning Methods for HER Data
From Data Extraction to Data Analytics
Hulin Wu, Jose Miguel Yamal, Ashraf Yaseen, Vahed Maroufy

Machine Learning in Medicine
Ayman El-Baz, Jasjit S. Suri

Advances in Mobile Health Technology
A Research Perspective
Sinjini Mitra

Advances in Mobile Health Technology

A Research Perspective

Sinjini Mitra

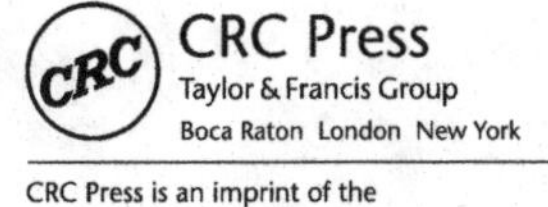

CRC Press is an imprint of the
Taylor & Francis Group, an **informa** business

First edition published 2023
by CRC Press
6000 Broken Sound Parkway NW, Suite 300, Boca Raton, FL 33487-2742

and by CRC Press
4 Park Square, Milton Park, Abingdon, Oxon, OX14 4RN

CRC Press is an imprint of Taylor & Francis Group, LLC

ISBN: 9781138369177 (hbk)
ISBN: 9781032372600 (pbk)
ISBN: 9780429428449 (ebk)

DOI: 10.1201/9780429428449

Typeset in Minion
by Newgen Publishing UK

Contents

Preface

MANAGING ONE'S OWN HEALTH IS MORE IMPORTANT THAN EVER NOW. The coronavirus or COVID-19 pandemic upended the lives of many and taught us the critical importance of taking care of one's health and wellness all over again. Technological advances coupled with advances in healthcare today have enabled the widespread growth of a new area called mobile health or mHealth, which has completely revolutionized how people envision healthcare today.

The World Health Organization (WHO) defines mHealth as 'medical and public health practice supported by mobile devices, such as mobile phones, patient monitoring devices, personal digital assistants (PDAs), and other wireless devices.'[1] The biggest potential of mHealth lies in its ability to help patients take control of their own health and being able to manage it in a sustained manner. This field has further grown with the emergence of wearable fitness trackers such as Fitbit, Apple Watches, etc., and mobile phone apps that not only help users keep track of their daily activities but also monitor key health indicators like blood pressure, heart rate, and blood oxygenation levels on a regular basis.

The aim of this book is to inform readers about the relatively modern technology of mHealth, from its history and evolution to the current state-of-the-art research developments and the underlying challenges related to privacy and security issues. Chapter 1 introduces the concept of mHealth, or mobile healthcare, and provides a broad overview of this technology. Chapter 2 includes a detailed overview of the history and evolution of various mHealth devices, which include both wearables and mobile health apps. Chapter 3 contains a detailed description of how mHealth technology works, and Chapter 4 presents a comprehensive review of research that has been done in the area of mobile health technology. Chapter 5 discusses the role of social media on personal health and wellness, while Chapter 6 addresses the topic of different issues and challenges that underlie this technology. Chapter 7 concludes the book with a glimpse of what the future holds for mobile healthcare technology.

Just as smartphones and tablet computers are rapidly becoming the dominant consumer computer platforms, mHealth technology is emerging as an integral part of consumer health and wellness management regimes. A recurring theme throughout this book is how the mHealth technology had enabled healthcare to be accessible to a wider section of the human population, especially to those living in developing countries and remote areas. The book's intended audience includes individuals interested in learning about mHealth and its contemporary applications, from students to researchers and practitioners working in this field. Both undergraduate and graduate students enrolled in college-level healthcare courses will find this book to be an especially useful companion and will be able to discover and explore novel research directions that will further enrich the field.

As modern technology and healthcare continue to make great strides, mHealth will also continue to grow and make stronger and stronger impacts on both individual and community health.

NOTE

1 World Health Organization *Frequently asked questions on Global Task Force on digital health for TB and its work.* [2017-02-27]. www.who.int/tb/areas-of-work/digital-health/faq/en/ *website*

Acknowledgments

Dr. Sinjini Mitra would like to thank her colleagues at the ISDS Department, Drs. Ester Gonzalez and Ofir Turel, for their early collaboration on mobile health research, which provided the motivation and foundation for this book. She also would like to acknowledge her graduate student, Shivani Agarwal, who conducted some preliminary research on mobile health. She is also grateful to Dr. Rahul Bhaskar, chair of the Information Systems and Decision Sciences (ISDS) Department, for his continual support throughout her career at CSUF. Last but not the least, she would like to extend her heartfelt appreciation to her middle-school-aged son, Soham Chakravarty, for developing an interest in research on mobile healthcare, particularly physical fitness trackers, of which he has been a long-time user, and contributing some background research on the topic that helped shape the book.

Finally, the author is thankful to the staff at Taylor & Francis, including Randi Cohen, senior acquisitions editor, and Talitha Todd-Duncan, for patiently working with us through the process of writing and publishing this book.

CHAPTER 1

Introduction to Mobile Healthcare (mHealth)

1.1 INTRODUCTION

Mobile healthcare, or m*Health* as it is commonly known, is gaining widespread popularity today. *Mobile healthcare* is a broad term typically used to describe the use of mobile technologies such as smartphones and tablet computers for health and wellness purposes. From text reminders to virtual clinic visits, mobile health is beginning to change the way healthcare is delivered and received. It offers not only improved efficiency via easy and convenient access but also has the potential to significantly improve the quality of outcomes, make healthcare more affordable by lowering costs, and increase the level of patient satisfaction [1].

Managing one's health is of utmost importance, and regular physical activity is one way to achieve this. This can help control or reduce weight, decrease the risk of certain diseases, and improve overall physical and mental health [2]. Today there is a wide variety of different mobile health devices and applications available to the general public. These include wearable fitness trackers, applications (or apps) for mobile phones, sleep monitors, heart rate meters, and exercise trackers. As newer mobile health devices are emerging in the market on a regular basis, the field is expanding with a market worth of U.S. $23 billion in 2017 and projected to grow at a CAGR (compound annual growth rate) of more than 35% over the next three years [3]. According to Zion market Research [4], the

DOI: 10.1201/9780429428449-1

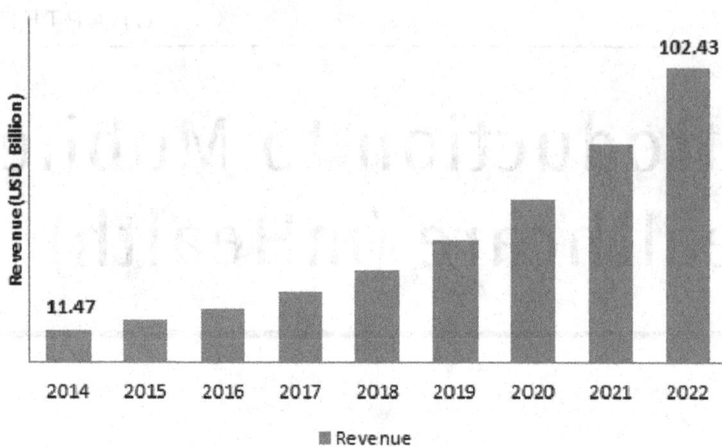

FIGURE 1.1 The growth of the mHealth market size, 2014–2022 [4].

global mHealth market is likely to cross U.S. $102.4 billion by the end of 2022 (Figure 1.1). The penetration of smartphones and the ongoing trend of wearable fitness devices, coupled with the rising awareness of the benefits of mobile healthcare technology, are among the key factors driving its market growth.

As mobile healthcare continues to grow, it becomes increasingly important to study its impact on consumers. Is it helping individuals to manage their health in a more effective way? What are the additional benefits is it offering compared to traditional healthcare services and delivery? These are some questions whose answers are crucial for the success and sustainability of mobile healthcare technology. According to [5], evidence supporting the effectiveness of mHealth in delivering high quality healthcare is limited. For some fields, the results are mixed while for others, no long-term studies exist in the literature at all. On the other hand, a recent survey of 600 global healthcare professionals in both private and public organizations of various sizes in Europe and the United States conducted by Vanson Bourne reports that mobile health devices and mHealth initiatives are strongly correlated with higher patient satisfaction scores [6]. They also found that the adoption of mobile technology in healthcare fields is very high, with 90% of organizations implementing or planning to implement a mHealth initiative. On the other hand, their confidence in their respective mHealth solutions that are deployed is quite low, about 48%, the top concern cited by respondents being security.

1.1.1 Fitness, Healthy Living, and Self-Health Management

Being and staying healthy is of utmost importance to an individual. Yet according to the U.S. Health and Human Services (HHS), over 78 million adults in the United States and 12.5 million (16.9%) children and adolescents are obese [7]. Recent reports also project that by 2030, 50% of U.S. adults will be obese [8]. These numbers have doubled over the past few decades and keep growing, which causes a lot of concern. There are several ways to take care of one's health and maintain a healthy lifestyle – namely, physical activity and exercise, maintaining proper diet and nutrition, maintaining a healthy weight, following healthy sleep patterns, reducing tobacco and alcohol use, and so on. (Figure 1.2 contains an infographic that illustrates these primary tools for a healthy lifestyle.) Of these, the most common means that people adopt to stay fit and healthy is physical activity or exercise. However, HHS reports that less than 5% of U.S. adults participate in at least 30 minutes of physical activity daily, and only one in three adults

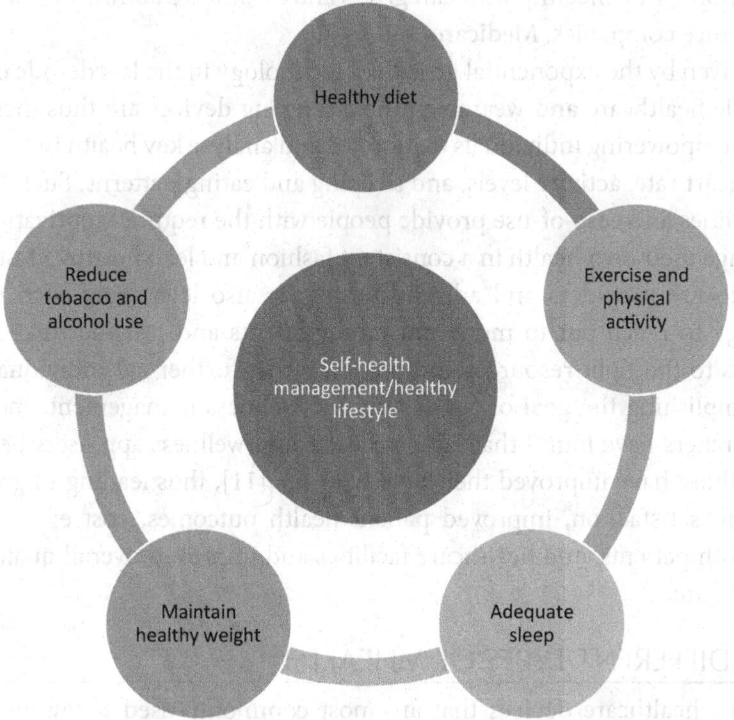

FIGURE 1.2 Infographic showing the primary aspects of self-health management that can help a person achieve and maintain a healthy lifestyle.

receives the recommended amount of physical activity in a week [9,10]. Lack of physical activity and exercise has been known to be a risk factor for cardiovascular diseases, type 2 diabetes, and certain types of cancer. Further, inactivity can lead to feelings of anxiety and depression that in turn may adversely affect ones' performance at work or in school and the quality of life in general. Leading a healthy lifestyle is thus associated with both short-term and long-term benefits, and therefore, there is a critical need to understand the barriers that people face in taking care of their own health and devise ways that can address these challenges, thus enabling them to lead a balanced and healthy lifestyle. Moreover, many individuals suffer from chronic health conditions such as diabetes, high blood pressure, joint pains like arthritis, and so on, which require constant monitoring and care. Self-health management tools are therefore essential in ensuring that such patients are able to live comfortably and receive the help they need and when they need it. This can be in the form of advice or medical attention from healthcare providers like doctors, nurses, and pharmacists, filling prescription, or connecting with caregivers and healthcare administrators like insurance companies, Medicare, and so on.

Driven by the exponential growth of technology in the last decade or so, mobile healthcare and wearable fitness tracking devices are thus increasingly empowering individuals to monitor and analyze key health indicators like heart rate, activity levels, and sleeping and eating patterns. Such functionalities and ease-of-use provide people with the required motivation to manage their own health in a consistent fashion and lead healthy lifestyles. Healthcare providers and administrators are also leveraging such technology to reach out to more and more patients and provide them with access to the right resources and materials that further aid individuals in accomplishing the goal of self-health and wellness management. Indeed, researchers have found that 96% of health and wellness app users believe that those have improved their quality of life [11], thus leading to greater patient satisfaction, improved patient health outcomes, cost efficiencies for both patients, and healthcare facilities and improved overall quality of healthcare.

1.2 DIFFERENT TYPES OF MHEALTH

Mobile healthcare devices that are most commonly used today by consumers can be divided into two groups based on type – (i) mobile device apps, and (ii) wearable fitness devices or trackers. The former are software applications on smartphones and/or tablets that have been developed to accomplish a certain purpose, such as track and monitor different kinds of physical activities and health conditions. These do not require the consumers to wear or carry any additional device. The latter, on the other hand, are devices that people have to wear particularly for tracking and monitoring their health and fitness activities. Although there may be other devices that fall under the broad umbrella of mobile health technology – such as patient monitoring devices (not necessarily connected to a computer or a mobile phone), mobile telemedicine and telecare devices, and so on – in this book we focus on the mobile apps and wearable fitness or activity devices that have became popular within the last decade or so. We provide a brief overview of these two broad types of mHealth in the next two subsections.

1.2.1 Mobile Device Apps

The pervasiveness of mobile devices and their increasing range of functionalities, such as the integration of different types of sensors, has enabled a wide spectrum of mobile applications that are transforming our daily lives. Similarly, new sensors capable of monitoring physiological data like body temperature, heart rate, and blood pressure, just to name a few, are gradually becoming more and more commonly available in today's mobile devices. Faster processors, improved memory, smaller batteries, and highly efficient open-source operating systems that perform complex functions have paved the way for the development of a flood of medical mobile device apps for both professional and personal use [12]. These have evolved from the basic health data monitoring capabilities to a multitude of more sophisticated health-related tasks. Because of the ease-of-use, which usually only requires a couple of taps on the mobile device and no additional cost involved, people are also increasingly using them various health-related activities. These not only help them manage their own health and wellness via regular monitoring but also complete common health activities and obtain relevant information and support about their own health conditions whenever they want. Figure 1.3 shows a typical interface of a health app on a modern smartphone.

The commonly available and used health or medical mobile apps can be divided into several broad groups as follows:

a) *Clinical assistance in diagnosis* – symptom checkers, digital imaging, health records check
b) *Remote patient health monitoring* – monitoring chronic conditions like cardiac health (heart rate, ECG), diabetes, oxygen levels, allergies

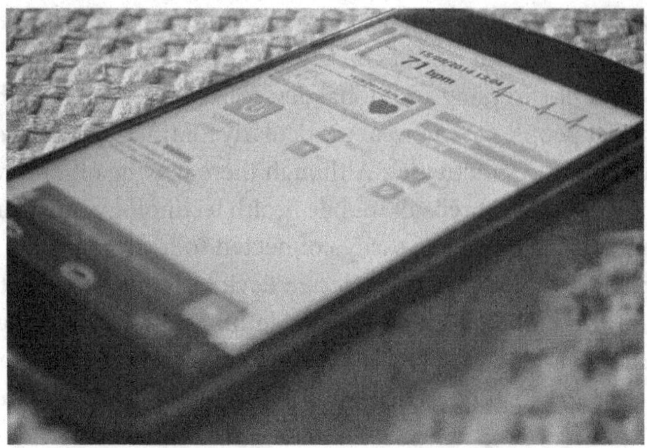

FIGURE 1.3 A typical mHealth app on a smartphone. (License: CC.)

c) *Reminders and alert systems* – doctor or clinic appointment reminders, prescription management, immunization reminders
d) *Healthy living* – diet monitoring and assistance, weight monitoring, exercise and fitness, healthy eating, pregnancy and baby development, sleep monitoring
e) *Education and awareness* – text messages sent directly to mobile phones to offer information about various subjects, including testing and treatment methods, availability of health services, and disease management (including mental health)
f) *Mobile social media* – capacity building to facilitate professional connectedness and to empower health workforce
g) *Other health services and delivery* – providing references to doctors hospitals, or pharmacies; making appointments to visit doctors, pharmacies or hospitals; scheduling surgeries

We discuss these individual health mobile apps in more details in Chapter 2.

1.2.2 Wearable Fitness Devices

Whether it is smart watches or fitness and health trackers, wearing technology is becoming a social standard. We have witnessed wearable technologies playing a major role in individual [13], organizational, and corporate wellness programs (e.g., Keller Williams) and intramural sports programs at colleges and universities (e.g., University of San Diego).

One in six consumers owns and uses wearable technology today [13]. Approximately 81.7 million United States adults were using wearable fitness trackers by the end of 2018 [14], and Gartner had projected that there will be 500 million wearable fitness devices in the hands of consumers by the year 2020 [15]. Because of this, it can be noted that there is a significant emphasis by the wearable industry to continue to promote and grow the market for these devices. Such devices typically consist of mini-computers that use sensors to gather different types of data about a person's activity and body ([16]). Accelerometers and altimeters are commonly used in such devices to measure steps, graph physical activity, calculate calorie breakdown, monitor heart rate, and record quality of sleep. Also, the altimeter enables users to get a higher level of accuracy in measuring the amount of physical activity when climbing stairs or hills. Algorithms translate these readings into helpful figures such as mileage or number of 'very active minutes.' Most wearable devices can be synced with a smartphone app or system, which analyze individual habits via 'data dashboards' – a collection of charts, graphs, and data tables. Moreover, one can share the results with others via a leaderboard that tap into social networking capabilities ([17]).

Some common wearable fitness tracking devices in use today include the Fitbit (several models such as Alta, Charge, Versa, and Ace for children), Apple Watch, Samsung Galaxy Watch, Nike Fuel Band, Garmin's Vivosmart and Vivosport, and the Huawei Band [18]. Of these, Fitbit, which debuted in the market in 2008 as a clip-on device, was one of the first fitness tracking devices to garner mainstream attention. We discuss various aspects of these devices in great details in several of the following chapters. Figure 1.4 shows a typical wearable fitness tracker on a person's wrist, and

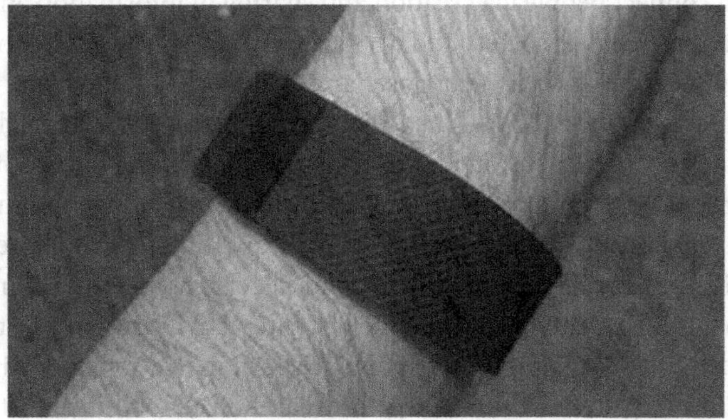

FIGURE 1.4 A typical wearable fitness device. (License: CC.)

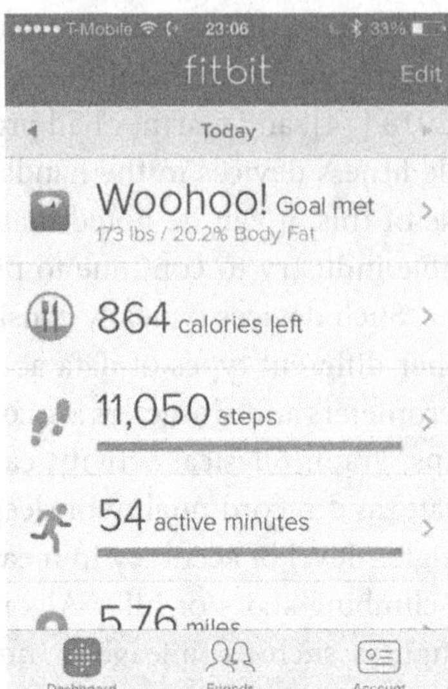

FIGURE 1.5 A typical mobile app interface of a fitness tracker (Fitbit). (License: CC.)

Figure 1.5 shows a typical interface of the mobile app for a common fitness tracker (Fitbit).

1.3 SOCIAL MEDIA AND MHEALTH

In this section, we provide a brief introduction to social media and its role in mHealth. This topic is discussed in more detail in Chapter 7.

1.3.1 Social Media

Social media, loosely defined as interactive computer-based technologies meant to connect people via creation and sharing of information and ideas [19], is a huge part of society today. Social media typically contains user-generated content such as text posts and comments, photos, and videos stored in a user's profile that is designed and maintained by a social media organization. Users then interact and communicate with each other and form groups with individuals they know, thus creating communities through social networking. Social media thus differs from traditional media like newspapers (paper-based) and television (electronic) in many ways, including quality, reach, frequency, interactivity, usability, and performance [20]. Some of the most popular social media websites with over 100 million registered users today are Facebook, YouTube, Instagram, Twitter, Tumblr, LinkedIn, Snapchat, Pinterest, and Reddit, to name a few.

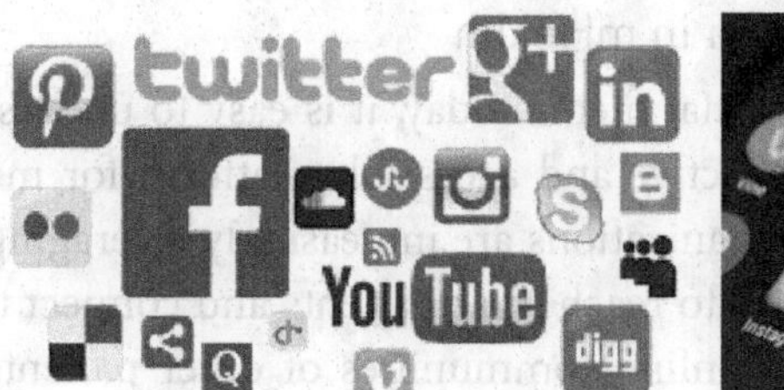

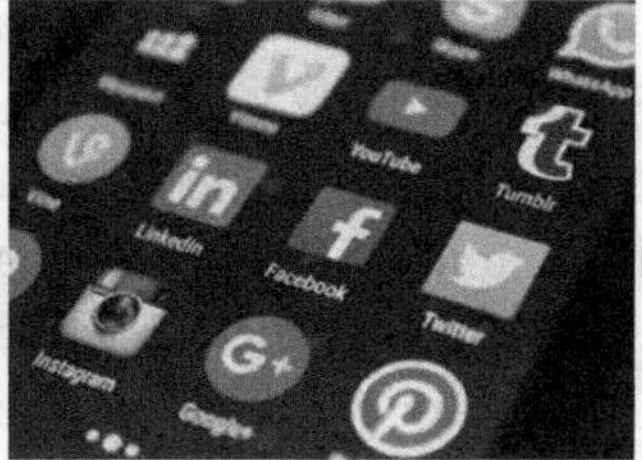

FIGURE 1.6 Examples of social media available today (left), social media apps on a mobile device (right). (License: CC.)

Of these, Facebook leads the way, with 2.27 billion users registered as of July 2018. Almost all of these websites can be accessed by an individual from any web-based technology, such as a computer desktop or laptops as well as a mobile device such as a smartphone or a tablet. Specific mobile applications or apps are also available on smartphones today to access such sites easily with the tap of a button, resulting in widespread access and use. Figure 1.6 shows a snapshot of these common social media sites and the corresponding apps available on a mobile device.

Researchers have reported both positive and negative impacts of social media use. Social media provides people with an easily accessible pathway to develop a sense of connectedness with different communities, real or online, and can be an effective tool for communication and marketing for different businesses and organizations. On the other hand, social media creates opportunities for online fraud (stealing of one's identity and data), online harassment, and cyber-bullying. According to a recent survey in the U.S., 69% of seventh grade students claim to have experienced cyber-bullying. All these lead to mental health issues, such as depression, anxiety, and stress that in turn lead to adverse effects on one's life and performance in school or at work. Moreover, studies have reported strong addictive behaviors among adolescents and youth regarding some types of social media usage, like gaming, that have been known to cause disruptions in sleep patterns, weight and exercise levels, and more prominently their academic performance. According to some recent research studies, long hours spent on mobile devices have shown a positive relationship with weight gain and decrease in physical activity levels in teenagers, while a strong negative relationship with GPA [21, 22]. It is thus probably advisable for everybody to use social media in a controlled manner so as to reap its benefits without affecting their own physical and mental health, and in particular, the usage by young people must be supervised and monitored by their parents.

1.3.2 The Role of Social Media in mHealth

Given the huge user base on social media today, it is easy to understand that it is able to provide an effective and accessible platform for mobile healthcare today. Healthcare organizations are increasingly leveraging the power of social networking sites to reach their patients and connect them with healthcare providers and online communities of other patients for different purposes, from helping them manage their own health to seek help and advice from both medical professionals and from other patients with similar health conditions and diagnoses. WebMD is a popular health information services website that publishes content regarding different aspects of healthcare as well as helping patients connect with doctors and other medical personnel. Towards the end of 2016, WebMD recorded an average of 179.5 million unique users per month and 3.63 billion page visits per quarter [23].

According to a Health Research Institute survey [16], 42% consumers are using social media today to access consumer reviews of treatments, physicians, and hospitals, and 20% have joined a health-related forum or community. However, the most interesting finding from the survey was that more than 80% of consumers in the age group 18–24 years use social media to use and share health information, and 40% mentioned that their healthcare decisions were influenced by social media. Moreover, more than 700 of the 5,000 U.S. hospitals have a social media presence to enhance their marketing efforts and establish effective communication with stakeholders.

Most fitness trackers like Fitbit provide the opportunity to connect with friends, family members, neighbors, and co-workers and share physical activity statistics with each other. Often, this is considered a way to obtain support in order to be successful in maintaining or achieving a healthy lifestyle. Competing with and receiving accolades for meeting activity goals can go a long way towards providing the motivation to an individual that is needed to keep him or her continuing to achieve health goals. Figure 1.7 below shows a typical mobile app dashboard of the popular fitness device Fitbit where the 'Friends' tab represents the social networking aspect.

Many corporate wellness programs are also encouraging their employees to use fitness trackers (often with incentives such as lowering the cost of the devices) in order to participate in individual and group tasks and challenges related to different types of physical activities for the purpose of maintaining a healthy lifestyle as well as lowering insurance costs for both the employer and the employees. Recent studies showed that two companies, Dayton

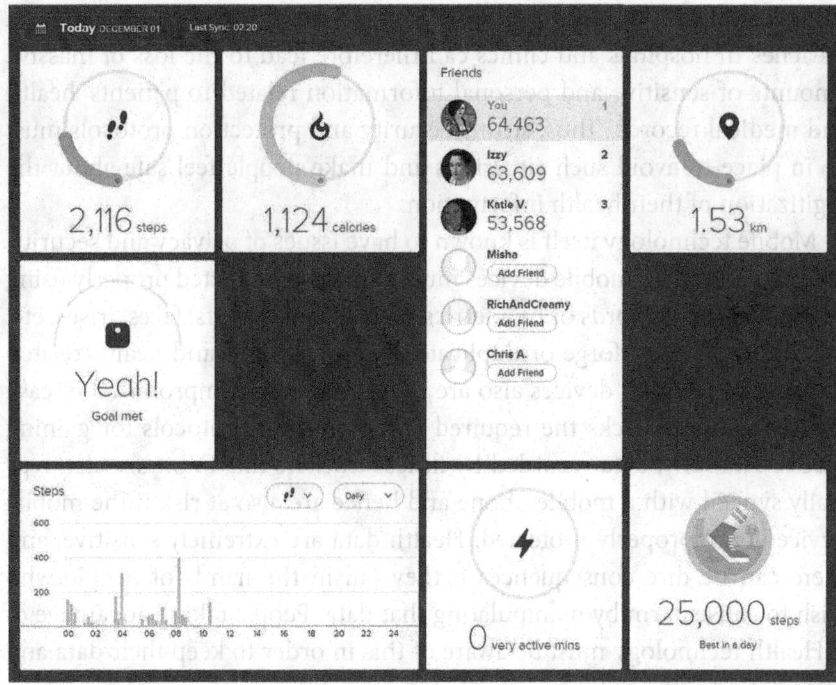

FIGURE 1.7 A typical dashboard interface of a fitness tracker that shows the 'social networking' aspect (Fitbit). (License: CC.)

Regional Transit Authority and Springbuk, deployed Fitbit as part of their organizational wellness programs and witnessed healthcare cost savings and improved health outcomes for their employees [25].

1.4 COMMON ISSUES AND CHALLENGES

Although many experts believe that mHealth technologies will play a major role in the healthcare industry in the future, their implementation is not without any issues and challenges that must be overcome successfully in order for a wider adoption of such strategies. We briefly outline some of the primary issues and challenges below and discuss this topic in more depth in Chapter 6.

1.4.1 Privacy and Security

Security in healthcare is a big challenge. The need to keep medical information of patients safe and thus avoid HIPAA (Healthcare Insurance Portability and Accountability Act) violations has become more complicated with the expansion of digital technology into healthcare. Data breaches in hospitals and clinics can therefore lead to the loss of massive amounts of sensitive and personal information related to patients' health and medical records. Thus, strong security and protection protocols must be in place to avoid such situations and make people feel safe about the digitization of their health information.

Mobile technology itself is known to have issues of privacy and security. The data stored on mobile devices must always be protected properly using either strong passwords or biometrics such as fingerprints, faces, irises, etc. that are difficult to forge or duplicate. So any medical and health-related data stored in those devices also are at risk of being compromised in case a person's phone lacks the required authentication protocols for gaining access. Similarly, data recorded by fitness trackers like Fitbit are also typically synced with a mobile phone and hence are also at risk if the mobile device is not properly protected. Health data are extremely sensitive, and there can be dire consequences if they fall in the hands of people who wish to cause harm by manipulating that data. People taking advantage of mHealth technology must be aware of this in order to keep their data and information safe.

Another potential issue with wearable fitness trackers is that such devices can be easily tracked with a portable scanner [26] that can divulge the wearer's location. Even if many of these fitness devices do not come with a GPS sensor built-in for tracking location, as soon as they are synced with a mobile device via Bluetooth, such location tracking can occur. This creates an additional hazard apart from the loss of personal information (say, your home or work address) and may even lead to criminal activities.

1.4.2 Organizational, Regulatory, and Support

The mHealth space today faces unique regulatory hurdles. mHealth companies need to be aware of and take into account the different health-related laws that are in effect in different states across the United States that include payment, medical board requirements, and prescription regulations [20]. Moreover, HIPAA laws are very stringent and require that all patients' medical and information must be collected and stored according to strict protocols that protect patients' rights to privacy and confidentiality. This applies to health data captured using mHealth devices.

Since mobile devices operate on wireless networks, having a strong and consistent signal is also essential for mHealth services to function properly.

This means that mHealth providers must work with the cell phone companies to ensure a reliable network that can support multiple kinds of devices and secure all information that is shared over it. This necessitates that both mHealth providers and wireless companies have a sufficient number of appropriate IT personnel or staff to help consumers troubleshoot any connectivity or access-related issues. This is extremely critical for the expansion and more widespread adoption of this technology to proceed smoothly.

1.4.3 Reliability and Accuracy of Data

The main challenge that is plaguing mHealth is the fact that while they provide a lot of data, their quality and reliability are often in question. First of all, not everybody records their data or syncs their fitness devices with their mobile devices on a regular basis, resulting in missing data. Further, there have been studies that have reported that some of the measurements recorded by mHealth devices are not even accurate. For example, [28] determined that some measurements (like step counts) may be more or less accurate and lie within 9% of the actual steps, whereas others (like distance traveled) may not be so. The study also showed that the faster the walking speed, the greater is the error for the distance measure. Similarly, calorie measurements have been shown to be barely rough estimates, and most heart-rate monitors and sleep monitors are not very reliable either [20].

Poor quality data are unable to yield valid results upon analysis, and hence no useful insights are obtained that are expected to be helpful to both healthcare providers and researchers. Doctors and physicians need accurate and consistently reliable data to offer suitable treatments for patients. On the other hand, research on the impact of fitness trackers and mHealth devices on people's health is sparse due to the problems with available data. Research is essential to understanding the full benefits of this technology that in turn can provide consumers with more confidence and motivation to use them for their personal health management. Therefore, steps must be undertaken to ensure that accurate, reliable, and valid data are collected from mHealth devices for in-depth research analyses. In this era of big data, sophisticated statistical and data mining tools are available to process, analyze, and interpret such health and fitness data, so there exists a definite need to leverage their capabilities to obtain the much-needed insights to guide future improvements to these products and improve the user experience at the same time.

1.5 ORGANIZATION AND LAYOUT OF THE BOOK

The book has seven chapters. Below is a brief outline of the remaining six chapters:

- ***Chapter 2*** provides an in-depth overview of the history and evolution of mHealth devices, starting with the pedometers, accelerometers to health and wellness apps on mobile devices (such as smartphones and tablet computers), followed by wearable fitness trackers and smartwatches like Fitbits, Apple Watch, and Garmin Vivoactive, to name a few. A timeline from the first-ever fitness tracking device to the current state-of-the-art is also included.
- ***Chapter 3*** contains a detailed description of how mHealth technology works. This includes functions and technologies underlying the sensors in the wearable devices, how fitness and health data are collected by these devices and the mHealth apps, and how these data and measurements help people track and manage their own health. The chapter concludes with some specific examples of the most popular mHealth devices today, such as Fitbit and Apple Watch.
- ***Chapter 4*** presents a comprehensive review of the existing literature on research that has been done in the area of mobile health technology to date, which covers published journal and conference papers, news articles, and research reports, among others. The areas that we will focus on include the impact of mHealth devices on different aspects of people's health, such as physical activity and fitness, sleep, weight loss, and healthy eating, as well as studies on the accuracy and reliability of these devices in tracking and monitoring health and fitness activities. The chapter includes the common research avenues explored thus far, issues and challenges on the way along with potential solutions, and trends and opportunities for future research in the area.
- ***Chapter 5*** focuses on the role of social media and social networking in promoting mHealth among consumers. The chapter starts with an overview of social media and its impact on personal health, what types of social media applications are associated today with fitness trackers and other mHealth technologies, and how people are using them today. The chapter concludes with a discussion about the various advantages and disadvantages of social media and its association with health and fitness, an overview of the current literature on the impact of social support and networking on people's motivation

and interest in adopting mHealth devices and the effect on health, and future trends and scope of research in this domain.

- ***Chapter 6*** addresses a very critical topic in all healthcare applications and particularly in mobile healthcare today – namely, the issues and challenges underlying the use of mHealth devices today. It particularly addresses topics such security, confidentiality, anonymity, and privacy; how common fitness devices ensure the security of the data collected; major pitfalls; and common problems and issues that are known and their effects on people's acceptance and adoption of such devices. The chapter ends with some broad guidelines about what steps might be undertaken by the manufacturers of mHealth devices to ensure their security, protect the users, and resolve the other issues and challenges.
- ***Chapter 7*** provides an overall summary of the entire book, along with a couple of mHealth case studies and an outline of the road ahead in terms of both research, practical applications, and utility of the mobile healthcare technology.

REFERENCES

1. Wagner, K. (2014). How Mobile Health is changing care delivery. Leadership, Link: www.hfma.org/leadership/mobilehealth/, published on November 4, 2014. Retrieved on February 24, 2019.
2. Centers for Disease Control and Prevention (2015). Physical activity and health. Link: www.cdc.gov/physicalactivity/basics/pa-health/. Retrieved on February 22, 2019.
3. Reuters (2017). mHealth Market Worth $23 Billion in 2017 and Estimated to Grow at a CAGR of more than 35% over the next three years. Link: www.reuters.com/brandfeatures/venture-capital/article?id=4640, published on April 18, 2017. Retrieved on February 24, 2019.
4. Zion Market Research (2018). mHealth Market to Branch out and Reach USD 102.32 Billion by 2022. Link: www.zionmarketresearch.com/news/global-mhealth-market, published on September 18, 2018. Retrieved on February 25, 2019.
5. Marcolino, M. S., Oliveira, J. Q. A., D'Agostino, M., Ribeiro, A. L., Alkmim, M. B. M., Novillo-Ortiz, D. (2018). The Impact of mHealth Interventions: Systematic Review of Systematic Reviews, *Journal of Medical Informatics Research (JMIR) mHealth and uHealth*, 6(1):e23.
6. Health, S. (2018). How do mHealth, Mobile Health devices Impact Patient Satisfaction? Patient Engagement health IT. Link: https://patientengagementhit.com/news/how-do-mhealth-mobile-health-devices-impact-patient-satisfaction, published on April 12, 2018. Retrieved on February 25, 2019.

7. Ogden, C.L., Carroll, M.D., Kit, B.K., Flegal, K.M. Prevalence of Obesity in the United States, 2009-2010. U.S. Centers for Disease Control and Prevention, National Center for Health Statistics Data Brief, January 2012. Link: www.cdc.gov/nchs/data/databriefs/db82.pdf – PDF, retrieved on March 27, 2019.
8. Wang, Y. Claire, McPherson, Klim, Marsh, Tim, Gortmaker, Steven L., Brown, Martin (2011). Health and Economic Burden of the Projected Obesity Trends in the USA and the UK. *The Lancet.*
9. U.S. Department of Agriculture. Dietary Guidelines for Americans, 2010. Available at: www.cnpp.usda.gov/dietaryguidelines.htm, retrieved on March 26, 2019.
10. U.S. Department of Health and Human Services. Healthy People 2010. Available at: www.cdc.gov/nchs/healthy_people/hp2010.htm, retrieved on March 27, 2019.
11. Clinician Today. How Technology Is Helping Health and Wellness Providers Promote Healthy Lifestyle Choices. Link: http://cliniciantoday.com/how-technology-is-helping-health-and-wellness-providers-promote-healthy-lifestyle-choices-infographic/, retrieved on March 27, 2019.
12. Ventola, C. L. (2014). Mobile Devices and Apps for Health Care Professionals: Uses and Benefits, *Pharmacy and Therapeutics*, 39(5): 356 – 364.
13. Piwek, L., Ellis, D.A., Andrews, S., Joinson, A. (2016). *The Rise of Consumer Health Wearables: Promises and Barriers. PLOS Medicine*. Published on February 2, 2016. https://doi.org/10.1371/journal.pmed.1001953.
14. Smith, C. (2016). Wearable Technology Statistics. Link: https://expandedramblings.com/index.php/wearables-statistics/, retrieved on December 15, 2018.
15. Levy, H. (2015). Wearable Technology Beyond Smartwatches. Smarter with Gartner, 2015. Link: www.gartner.com/smarterwithgartner/wearable-technology-beyond-smartwatches-3/, published on October 21, 2015. Retrieved on February 25, 2019.
16. Roberts, A. (2019). The Best Fitness Trackers, WireCutter review, link: https://thewirecutter.com/reviews/the-best-fitness-trackers/, published on February 8, 2019. Retrieved on February 25, 2019.
17. CNN Report (2013). Fitness tools that ta the power of your friends. Link: www.cnn.com/2013/06/03/tech/mobile/fitness-gadgets-motivation/ – Fitness Studies get Social, published on June 3, 2013. Retrieved March 26, 2015.
18. McGuire, J. (2021). Best fitness trackers in 2021: Top activity bands from Fitbit, Garmin and more, Tom's guide, Link: www.tomsguide.com/us/best-fitness-trackers,review-2066.html, published on November 30, 2021. Retrieved on November 30, 2021.
19. Social media Wikipedia page: https://en.wikipedia.org/wiki/Social_media, retrieved on February 27, 2019.

20. Agichtein, E., Castillo, C., Donato, D., Gionis, A., Mishne, G. (2008). Finding high-quality content in social media, *WISDOM – Proceedings of the 2008 International Conference on Web Search and Data Mining*: 183–193.
21. Rafla, M., Carson, N. J., Dejong, S. M. (2014). Adolescents and the Internet: What Mental Health Clinicians Need to Know, *Current Psychiatry Reports*, 16 (9): 472. doi:10.1007/s11920-014-0472-x PMID 25070673.
22. Junco, R. (2012). Too Much Face and Not Enough Books: The relationship between multiple indices of Facebook use and academic performance. *Computers in Human Behavior*. 28(1):187–198.
23. WebMD Wikipedia page: https://en.wikipedia.org/wiki/WebMD, retrieved of February 27, 2019.
24. Innovatemedtech (2019). Social Media in Healthcare. Link: https://innovatemedtec.com/digital-health/health-social-media-in-healthcare, retrieved on February 27, 2019.
25. Landi, H. (2016). Study: Fitbit Corporate Wellness Programs cut Employer Healthcare Costs, *Healthcare Innovation*. Link: www.hcinnovationgroup.com/population-health-management/mobile-health-mhealth/news/13027550/study-fitbit-corporate-wellness-programs-cut-employer-healthcare-costs, published on October 5, 2016. Retrieved on February 27, 2019.
26. Eadicicco, L. (2014). A new wave of gadgets can collect your personal information like never before, *Business Insider*, link: www.businessinsider.com.au/privacy-fitness-trackers-smartwatches-2014-10, published on October 10, 2014. Retrieved on September 12, 2017.
27. Mcaskill, R. (2015). The Challenges of implementing mHealth, *mHealth Intelligence*, link: https://mhealthintelligence.com/news/the-challenges-of-implementing-mhealth, published on February 9, 2015. Retrieved on February 27, 2019.
28. Lee, J. M., Kim, Y., Welk, G. J. (2014). Validity of consumer-based physical activity monitors, *Medicine and Science in Sports and Exercise*, 46(9): 1840–1848.

CHAPTER 2

The Evolution and History of mHealth and Fitness Trackers

2.1 INTRODUCTION

The field of mobile health, or mHealth technology, in recent years has emerged and grown exponentially worldwide for both developed and developing countries, stemming primarily from the rapid rise of mobile phone penetration. The underlying objective of this technology was to provide access to healthcare to a larger segment of the population as well as improve the capacity of health systems to provide quality healthcare to patients. However, with further advancement of technology and increasing awareness of healthy living among the general public, mHealth has evolved significantly to encompass tools that help individuals monitor their exercise and physical activity levels, food and water intake, calories burned, sleep patterns, etc., and thus enable them to lead healthy lifestyle by managing their own well-being in a very cost-effective and convenient manner.

The most popular mobile healthcare devices used by consumers today can be categorized into two groups based on type – (i) mobile device health and wellness apps, and (ii) wearable fitness (or activity) trackers or devices. In this chapter we describe these different mHealth devices and their applications, as well as provide background on the history and evolution of these types of devices, starting from the very first ones to the current

DOI: 10.1201/9780429428449-2

state-of-the art. The chapter is organized as follows. We start with an overview of the mobile device health apps in Section 2.2, followed by the wearable fitness devices in Section 2.3. Section 2.4 briefly discusses the most popular devices today such as Fitbits and Apple Watches, among others, and finally we conclude in Section 2.5 with an outline of the future this technology.

2.2 MOBILE DEVICE HEALTH APPS

Mobile health or medical applications (apps) are defined by the U.S. Food and Drug Administration (FDA) [1] as 'software on a mobile device that function as an accessory to a regulated medical device or transform a platform into a regulated medical device.' In other words, these apps can help patients manage their own health and wellness, promote healthy living, and gain access to useful information when and where they need it. Moreover, such apps can be used for remote patient monitoring, medical consultations, and disease management, thus helping healthcare practitioners facilitate and improve patient care. Hence, these tools are being adopted almost as quickly as they can be developed by healthcare professionals, consumers, and patients because of their accessibility and ease-of-use. Figure 2.1 shows a snapshot of some existing health apps on an Apple iPhone.

According to a recent report [2], 325,000 mobile health and wellness apps were available at the end of the year 2017, with the addition of around

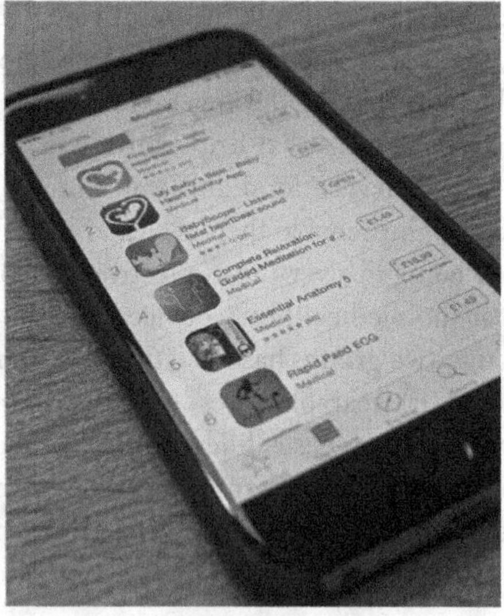

FIGURE 2.1 Some mHealth apps on an iPhone. (License: CC.)

78,000 new apps just in the year 2017, which shows a growth of 25%. Currently, Android leads this area, with 158,000 health-related apps available on the Google Play Store, followed by Apple, which also has about 152,000. Other mobile platforms like Blackberry, Microsoft Windows, and Amazon also offer about 10,000–15,000 mHealth apps. A report published by Zion Market Research [3] states that the global mHealth apps market that was valued at USD 8 billion is projected to generate around USD 111.1 billion by the year 2025 at a CAGR (Compound Annual Growth Rate) of 32.8% between 2019 and 2025. So over time, it is estimated that both the availability and adoption of mobile health apps will continue its upward growth trend.

2.2.1 Mobile Health Apps in the Global Market Today

The global mobile health apps market is segmented by region. In 2017, North America accounted for about 40% of the global mHealth apps market and had the largest market share in terms of revenue [3]. This is in part fueled by the presence of advanced healthcare infrastructure in the U.S. and Canada and the growing prevalence of various chronic diseases, such as diabetes, hypertension, respiratory diseases, and cancer, that require regular monitoring and management. Among the U.S. and Canada, the U.S. leads the market share in mHealth apps.

Next is Europe in terms of the size of the mHealth apps market, with Germany holding the largest revenue share, about 30%, followed by France and the UK. The increasing adoption of mHealth apps, developed healthcare systems, and the high focus on precision and personalized medicine are the main drivers of the growth of the European mHealth apps market and revenue.

In the Asia-Pacific region, the mHealth apps market has started blooming in the last few years and is likely to register the highest CAGR between 2019 and 2025. This is primarily owing to the high prevalence of chronic diseases such as arthritis and cardiovascular diseases, large population size, the need to reduce healthcare costs, as well as the widespread adoption of smartphones among the masses. The Asian countries with the most mHealth apps in use today are India, China, and Japan.

The growth of the mHealth apps market is expected to be the slowest for Africa and the Middle East. This is attributed to reasons such as the lack of advanced healthcare amenities and infrastructure and low awareness of health and wellness among the general population. South America is anticipated to make moderate growth in the mHealth apps market in the near future, driven by the proliferation of smartphone technology and the adoption of wearable fitness devices. Brazil leads the Latin America region today in terms of the mobile health apps market share and revenue.

2.2.2 Evolution of Mobile Health Apps

The emergence of mobile health apps in the market was spearheaded by the revolution of smartphone technology that officially started with the Apple's first iPhone in 2007. Although smartphones were launched as early as in the 1990s, with IBM's 'Simon,' followed by the Ericsson R380 in 2000 and Kyocera 6035 in 2001, these were basically hybrid devices that integrated the functionalities of a Personal Digital Assistant (PDA) with basic phone hardware [4]. The iPhone was the first of its kind that was designed with a capacitive touchscreen that supported multi-touch gestures and interactions, such as zooming in photos and websites, and very quickly entered the mainstream of consumer use. As of 2010, there were already 5,820 apps within the health and wellness categories on smartphones [5]. This number grew very quickly to more than 17,000 by the end of the year 2013, mostly focused on consumers. In 2020, there were 45,478 healthcare apps available on the Apple iOS platform [6] and 43,285 on Android devices [7].

With the availability of so many health apps on different mobile platforms, consumers have a choice to select the ones that are useful to them. There are several factors that drive consumer choices in this regard, particularly for continual or sustained use over a long period of time. According to [8], some key factors that influence an users' decision to adopt a certain health app are the design and interface that facilitate ease-of-use and navigation, reliability, and accuracy of information contained in or presented by those apps, alignment with one's personal health goal management, and actionable recommendations, among others. According to research conducted by Accenture, consumer use of mobile health apps is rising, driven by the explosive growth in mobile technology usage in the current decade [8] along with other factors, such as new business models and new workflows and policies that are quickly transforming the landscape of healthcare across different nations. About 85% of people today in the United States own a smartphone, up from just 35% in 2011 (as per a Pew Research Center report, [9]), and about 97% own a mobile phone of some kind. The number of mHealth app downloads worldwide thus increased very rapidly from 1.7 billion in 2013 to 3.7 billion in 2017 (a 118% growth over the period of 5 years). Moreover, surveys mention that nearly 80% of consumers prefer and use mHealth apps on their mobile devices today [8]. According to an mHealth Economics 2017 study [10], the top three fields with the best market potential for mobile health solutions are in the areas of disease management, particularly, diabetes, obesity, and depression. Although these therapy fields have a large market potential, the market penetration is generally low.

The FDA encourages the development of mobile health apps that promise to improve the quality of healthcare today in the United States and provide consumers and healthcare professionals with valuable health-related and medical information. It issued the '*Policy for Device Software Functions and Mobile Medical Applications Guidance*' first in 2013 with the goal of informing manufacturers of software devices and applications about their own regulatory authorities regarding the selection of such applications for use on mobile and other platforms. This policy was further updated in 2015 and 2019.

2.2.3 Types of Mobile Health Apps

The global mHealth apps market is segmented based on type. Broadly, such apps can be divided into two groups, namely, *healthcare apps* (also called *wellness* apps) and *medical apps*. Of these, healthcare apps are the most widely adopted and hence have the greatest market share. Medical apps are usually used by doctors and hence are fewer in number. Healthcare or wellness apps are used by individuals, from regular health monitoring to finding doctors and hospitals. The commonly available and used health or medical mobile apps can be divided into several broad groups based on functionality as follows:

a) *Clinical assistance in diagnosis* – symptom checkers to diagnose diseases and other health issues, manage digital imaging, and check health records. 'MyScripps' is an app that helps patients access their health and medical information remotely at any time, as well as allow them to check symptoms for a potential disease or health condition.
b) *Remote patient health monitoring and managing chronic conditions* – managing chronic conditions like cardiac health (heart rate, ECG), diabetes, oxygen levels, and allergies, and monitoring and managing regular health conditions related to pre-natal care, cancer care, ophthalmology, infectious disease care, and mental health issues [1]. 'Pain Coach' by WebMD is an app that can help measure pain levels

associated with a chronic condition, and seek treatments when needed, etc. 'Glucose Buddy' is a diabetes management app that allows users to manually log glucose numbers, carb consumption, insulin dosages, and activity so as to keep track of them. Similarly, 'Healthy Heart 2' is an app for recording blood pressure, cholesterol levels, pulse, and medications, etc. which can be shared with physicians periodically.

c) *Remote physician consultation* – online medical help-seeking and consulting with a professional. 'Dr. Now' and 'Doctor on Demand' are some medical apps where somebody can connect to a doctor online for professional consultation. Similarly, 'MeMD' is an app that provides online medical consultations with doctors, nurse practitioners, and physician assistants in the U.S., including obtaining certain prescriptions (as permitted by state laws) and addressing certain mental health issues such as anxiety, depression, abuse, addiction, panic attacks, and so on.

d) *Reminders and alert systems* – doctor or clinic appointment reminders, prescription management, immunization reminders, epidemic outbreak alerts.

e) *Healthy living* – diet monitoring and assistance, weight monitoring, exercise and fitness, healthy eating, pregnancy and baby development, sleep monitoring.

f) *Education and awareness* – text messages sent directly to mobile phones or information available on websites about various medical and health-related subjects, including testing and treatment methods, drug information, availability of health services, and disease management (including mental health). The 'CDC mobile app' provides a full library of medical information, access to journals, disease tracking information, public health blogs, and many more resources for consumers.

g) *Mobile social media* – capacity building to facilitate professional connectedness for patients as well as community building among patients and families of patients who suffer from similar health and/or chronic conditions to exchange and share information, advice, and experiences. 'LivingWith' is a health app that can help cancer patients to connect with their friends and family, find relevant information about a specific type of cancer, read inspirational patient stories, and connect with different advocacy groups.

h) *Other health services and delivery* – providing references to doctors, hospitals, or pharmacies; making appointments to visit a doctor, pharmacy, or hospital; scheduling tests and surgeries. MyChart is one of the leading mHealth apps today for patients to schedule appointments and also to access their health records remotely.

i) *Health insurance and claims processing* – providing resources to patients about their insurance coverage and benefits and facilitating a unified electronic claim process that includes submission and status tracking. 'Covered California' is an excellent example of a mobile insurance app.

Not only patients but clinicians and physicians, too, now are realizing the benefits of mobile health technology that is very easily accessible through their own smart mobile devices like cell phones and tablets. The most commonly used medical apps adopted by healthcare professionals today include the following:

a) *Epocrates* – often considered as the 'gold standard' for medical apps, Epocrates help doctors to find drug-related information, offer drug specifications and recommendations to patients, find providers and referrals for patients quickly, and also calculate some patient measurements like BMI (Body mass index) for a quick evaluation.

b) *Medscape* – this app provides doctors with information about drug doses and adverse drug combinations and enables discussions among medical professionals and the sharing of advice and experiences with different aspects of healthcare, access to medical updates, and a plethora of other health and medical resources.

c) *UpToDate* – this app helps medical professionals to stay up to date with medical advances and updates and answers to medical questions anywhere and anytime. It is thus considered a continuing education resource by way of providing an extensive repository of data and information along with medical calculators and communication functions.

d) *Skyscape* – this app provides physicians, nurses and even medical students with access to over 400 resources from leading publishers, authors, and medical societies regarding drug information (both brands and generics), dose calculators and interactions, along with important clinical information to help with diagnosis of diseases and disorders based on symptoms.

e) *Pepid* – this app is a premium diagnostic one as it helps medical personnel to detect diseases and disorders based on symptoms that a patient might be experience at a certain point of time. It thus helps such individuals to visualize a wide range of possible outcomes and make the right point-of-care decisions.

Apart from these popular and common ones, there are several others available today on both the Apple iOS and Android platforms, such as *Read by QxMD*[1] and *MedPage Today*,[2] which provide access to medical journals through different sources like PubMed and medical news, and *Appointik*[3] and *Kareo*,[4] which can be used by certain medical professionals for administrative purposes such as managing billing and marketing endeavors for their practices and setting up and managing appointments with patients and other healthcare professionals or stakeholders (such as insurers, etc.).

Some common health and fitness mobile apps that are meant to encourage and support healthy living and lifestyle are outlined below [11]:

a) *Noom*[5] – this is a popular app today that helps individuals with weight loss. It helps to train one's body into adopting healthier habits. Experts and coaches are also available to provide help to set personal achievable goals and attain them.

b) *Lifesum* – this app is meant to provide help with diet for people who want to lose weight. It mainly focuses on tracking calories and provides input about what changes to make in order to achieve one's weight goals.

c) *FitStar* – this app provides a set of fitness tracking tools, video demonstrations, and expert coaching tips to help people get fit anytime, anywhere (works with iPhone and iPad). Their tools are adaptive and get more advanced as someone makes progress. The user can provide feedback to the app, which is used to tailor each routine to their needs and match their fitness levels. It can also be customized to a person's strength and stamina.

d) *Pedometer++* – This is an iPhone app that keeps track of one's daily and weekly steps, without losing any battery. The progress can be viewed on the app itself or can be synced with an Apple Watch.

e) *Wakeout* – This app is one of the most popular apps on iPhone and has over 1,000 exercises that one can choose from and start anytime. The app can even remind users if they are sitting for too long as well.

f) *Sweat* – This app is made for women and offers many different recipes and programs to help achieve one's health and fitness goals. There is a program where the user can get his/her boost of confidence in the weight rooms of a gym and also has access to personal trainers and coaches.

2.3 WEARABLE FITNESS DEVICES

Wearable fitness devices or activity trackers are external devices attached to an individual for the purpose of tracking and measuring different physiological parameters of the body. These devices come in different sizes and shapes and are equipped with some overall basic functions (such as number of steps, distance walked or run, active minutes, etc.) along with additional features (such as calorie consumption, amount of sleep, heartbeat monitoring, etc.) in some of them. Most of the modern devices available today are water-resistant and can track exercise activity while swimming and while participating in other water sports like diving, water polo, etc. These are often termed as 'wearable computers' and are synced wirelessly usually to a computer or a smartphone for constant data tracking and monitoring. Although they are sometimes referred to as 'technology fads,' some health benefits have led to the widespread adoption of fitness trackers by general populations worldwide. As technology continues to expand, we take a look at how all these started and where we are at right now in the next sections.

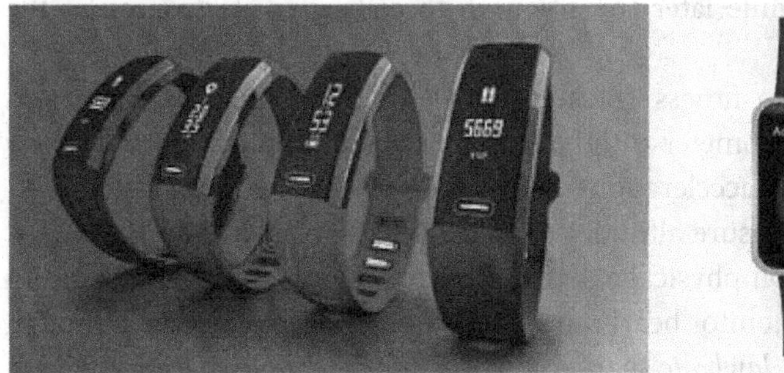

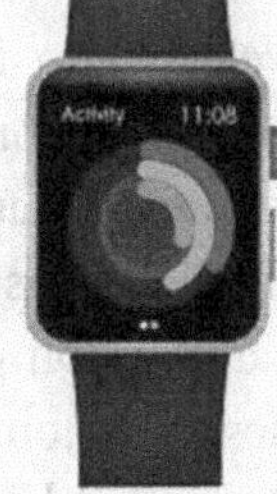

FIGURE 2.2 Some common fitness trackers and a smartwatch in use today. (License: CC.)

2.3.1 Evolution of Fitness Trackers

Improvements and innovations in technology in the late 20th and early 21st centuries are the main driving forces behind the automation of health and fitness tracking and their integration with easily wearable equipment. Some early examples include wristwatch-sized computers that could be mounted on a bicycle handlebar called *cyclocomputers* (or simply, 'bicycle computers') and could calculate trip information such as speed, duration and distance. It was invented in 1895 by Curtis H. Veeder and was available in the early 1900s.

Fitness or activity trackers have come a long way since then, but according to some sources [12], the history of these devices dates all the way back to the 1700s. In 1780 Abraham-Louis Perrelet, a Swiss horologist and inventor, created the first *pedometer.* It was capable of measuring steps and distance while walking. Thomas Jefferson introduced the first mechanical pedometer in the United States shortly afterwards, although its popularity did not take off till the 1930s and was popular mostly among long-distance walkers and did not reach the general population. The modern fitness tracker as we know today was first marketed in 1965 in Japan and was known as *Manpo-kei* (meaning '10,000 steps meter' in Japanese) which claimed that 10,000 steps per day was ideal for maintaining a healthy body. This device was invented by Dr. Yoshiro Hatano while researching ways to combat obesity.

Since the 1960s, fitness tracking devices and their underlying technology has evolved at a rapid pace. In 1981, wearable heart-rate monitors integrated in Polar watches were available for athletes (Polar RS800 model). This was followed by fitness tracking devices and heart-rate monitoring being integrated with commercial-grade fitness equipment in gyms and fitness centers, while later transitioning to consumer electronics by the early 2000s.

Most electronic fitness trackers today are fundamentally improved versions of the pedometer with built-in advanced tools like *accelerometers* (tools that measure acceleration or the rate of change of velocity) and *altimeter* (tools that measure altitude) to calculate distance covered (in miles), compare and graph physical activity, measure calorie expenditure, and in some cases also monitor heart rates, exercise, and sleep patterns. Although a company called *Jawbone* sparked the wearable technology industry with its *Up24* activity tracker in 2011, the mainstream revolution in this domain in the United States (and later across the rest of the world) was spearheaded by *Fitbit*, a company founded in Delaware in 2007 (formerly named *Healthy Metrics Research*). *Fitbit* introduced its first activity tracker in 2009 that could be clipped to the waist, with more modern and diverse designs appearing in the market at a rapid pace after that such as those with wrist bands (*Fitbit Flex, Fitbit Alta,*· *Fitbit Charge, Fitbit Inspire,* etc.) and, even more recently, smartwatches (*Fitbit Blaze, Fitbit Versa, Fitbit Ionic, Fitbit Sense*, etc.). This was also the first company to produce a fitness tracker that was specifically meant for children aged eight and above (*Fitbit Ace*) in 2018. Some of the older Fitbit models have now been retired, but it is still the most popular fitness tracking device on the market today. We discuss the different models and their timelines in more detail in the next section.

In 2010, Nike and Apple together developed the *Nike+iPod* activity tracker that could be embedded or attached to shoes to track activity via the iPod Nano. Following this trend, companies like Samsung (*Samsung Gear Fit*), Garmin (*Vivosmart and Vivofit*), TomTom (*TomTom Touch*), Nike (*FuelBand*), and so on, have released wearable fitness tracking devices in the market over the last five years. Some international vendors of wearable technology include Chinese technology companies *Xiaomi* and *Huawei*, both of whose products are available in the U.S. markets as well. A more recent innovation in this domain of wearable fitness technology is the *Oura ring* (a 'smart ring') that can be worn on a finger and used to track activity and sleep. One interesting feature of this device that is different from the other mainstream fitness trackers is its ability to read the user's temperature.

In 2012, Pebble Technology first introduced a smartwatch whose development was propelled by a $10.3 million funding through a Kickstarter campaign [13]. Although this device has now been discontinued, the smartwatch market has grown tremendously and is projected to overtake that of the regular wearables soon. Leading the pack here is Apple, which introduced the *iWatch* or the *Apple Watch* for the first time in April 2015. Soon after its release, it became the best-selling wearable device, with 4.2 million sales recorded only in the second quarter of the fiscal year 2015. Since then, a new version or series has been introduced every year, with the latest model being the Series 5 released on September 20, 2019. We discuss this device in more details along with a timeline in the next section. At present, Samsung (*Samsung Galaxy Watch*), Fitbit, (*Surge, Versa, Ionic, etc.*),

TABLE 2.1 A chronology of the most popular modern fitness trackers and smart watches

Fitness tracking device	Type of device	Date released[6]
First Pedometer	Pedometer	1780s
Manpo-kei (Japan)	Pedometer	1965
Polar watch	Smartwatch	1981
Fitbit 'Fit'	Standalone tracker (waist clip)	2009
Jawbone Up24	Standalone tracker	2011
Pebble smartwatch	Smartwatch	2012
Nike Fuelband	Standalone tracker	2012
Fitbit	Standalone tracker (wristband)	2013
Fitbit Surge	Smartwatch	2014
Xiaomi Mi Smart band	Standalone tracker	2014
Garmin Vivofit	Standalone tracker	2014
Garmin Vivoactive	Smartwatch	2014
Samsung Gear Fit	Standalone tracker	2014
Huawei Honor Band	Standalone tracker	2015
Apple Watch	Smartwatch	2015
Huawei Watch	Smartwatch	2015
TomTom Touch	Standalone tracker	2016
Samsung Galaxy Watch	Smartwatch	2018
Verizon GizmoWatch	Smartwatch	2018
Xiaomi Amazfit Bip	Smartwatch	2020

Garmin (*Vivoactive*), Xiaomi (*Amazfit Bip*), Verizon (*GizmoWatch* meant for kids aged 3–11 years), and Huawei (*Huawei Watch*) all have produced smartwatches that are available to consumers for purchase and are potential competitors of the Apple Watch.

Table 2.1 provides a chronology of the most popular modern fitness trackers (including smart watches) produced by the major vendors as they appeared on the market. Note that most vendors have multiple products in each format or category (e.g., Flex, Alta, Charge, etc., are different standalone trackers produced by Fitbit) and multiple versions of each model (e.g., Apple Watch Series 3, 4, 5, etc.) that are released sequentially, which we do not address here specifically.

Table 2A.1 (Appendix) outlines the different models and versions of these well-known standalone fitness trackers and smartwatches produced by the top vendors including both the state-of-the-art and older models (some of which may have been retired). This clearly shows how fast this technology is changing and improving almost on a daily basis and holds enormous potential for the future as well.

2.4 COMMON FITNESS TRACKERS

According to many reports, the best-selling and hence most popular fitness trackers are the ones produced by Fitbit [14]. Fitbit has several models that are suitable for a wide section of the general population today, including children. Similarly, among smartwatches, Apple Watch, produced by Apple Inc., is the most popular model today. In this section, we briefly review the evolution of these two products over the years since they were first launched.

2.4.1 Fitbit

As mentioned briefly earlier, Fitbit started the wearable technology trend with its first wristband-based fitness or activity tracker called Fitbit Flex in 2013. According to a report published on March 10, 2020, Fitbit is currently the fifth largest wearable technology company based on shipments in 2019 with an 14.8% annual growth, behind Xiaomi and Apple [15]. It is estimated that Fitbit sales have reached 100 million, with 28 million users worldwide. Starting with the first tracker invented in 2009 as a waist clip, its models and designs have diversified considerably, with newer features incorporated on a continual basis over the past decade. We summarize below all the products that have been released by Fitbit over the years to facilitate an easy overview of how the brand evolved:

- *Clip-on trackers like Fit (or Classic), Fitbit Ultra, Fitbit One, and Fitbit Zip* – released between 2009 and 2012, and discontinued at this time. They could be clipped on the waist or the pocket of a user. The two latter models had syncing capabilities with mobile devices to track data over time.
- *Fitbit Flex* – the first wristband tracker from Fitbit was introduced in 2013. It tracked activities and movements and also sleep patterns. It could be paired with a smartphone and also offered social networking capabilities to connect to friends and family to share activity statistics. This product has been discontinued now.
- *Fitbit Flex 2* – an improvement over the Fitbit Flex released in 2016 that was capable of tracking swimming. This product has been discontinued now.
- *Fitbit Force* – this model, released in October 2013, had an OLED display that showed time and daily activity. However, owing to some

concerns from users regarding allergic skin reactions, the product was recalled and ultimately discontinued.

- *Fitbit Charge and Fitbit Charge 2* – these products were introduced in 2014 and 2015, respectively, to replace the Fitbit Force but have since been discontinued and replaced by newer models. These models were able to track upward movement (such as climbing of stairs). The Charge 2 had a slightly larger screen than the Charge.
- *Fitbit Charge HR* – released in 2015, this product was the first one in the Fitbit line to integrate a heart-rate monitor. This model has also been discontinued now.
- *Fitbit Alta and Fitbit Alta HR* – introduced in 2016 and 2017, these were new models with a different look than the Fitbit Charge designs, with an improved capacity to track the different stages of sleep. The latter also included a heart-rate monitor. Both models are now discontinued.
- *Fitbit Charge 3* – released in October 2018, this model features a heart-rate tracker along with an oxygen saturation sensor and an improved sleep tracker. Later, 'Fitbit Pay' was also integrated with this model. It is currently still available in the market.
- *Fitbit Inspire and Fitbit Inspire HR* – newer models introduced in February 2019 and currently still being produced. These arrived in the market as a replacement for Fitbit Charge 2. The HR model includes heart-rate monitoring.
- *Fitbit Charge 4* – released in March 2020, this model has advanced features compared to the Fitbit Charge 3 that include in-built GPS, Spotify controls (to play music), Active Zone Minutes, and Fitbit Pay support.
- *Fitbit Luxe* – released in April 2021, it is very similar to Fitbit Inspire 2. It is mainly targeted towards female users and has a fashionable look with a color touchscreen display. Features include heart-rate monitoring, sleep monitoring, and female health tracking.
- *Fitbit Charge 5* – currently the state-of-the-art model from Fitbit released in September 2021, it is an upgraded version of the Fitbit Charge 4 and has the capabilities to monitor the user's heart health, track stress, and the add-on ability to track your body to carry out the required workouts.

- *Fitbit Ace and Fitbit Ace 2* – the first activity trackers specifically meant for kids, Ace was released in 2018 for children aged eight and above. It has been discontinued now and has been replaced by the Ace 2 since 2019, which is meant for kids aged six and above.

Below is a summary of the different smartwatches manufactured by Fitbit, starting with the first one from over six years back, in 2014:

- *Fitbit Surge* – released in 2014, this was a smartwatch and a fitness tracker. It also had a heart-rate monitor and could track pace, distance and elevation using an in-built GPS. It could also display incoming text and phone calls from a connected mobile phone. This model has now been discontinued.
- *Fitbit Blaze* – released in 2016, this model was introduced to compete with the Apple Watch, which was launched in 2015. For the first time, this had a colored touchscreen and advanced features that could be used in conjunction with the paired smartphone. This model has now been discontinued.
- *Fitbit Ionic* – released in 2017, this model replaced the Fitbit Blaze with several design options (for different looks like a sports watch, for example) and new features to continue the competition with the newer Apple Watch Series 3.
- *Fitbit Versa, Fitbit Versa 2, and Fitbit Versa 3* – released in 2018, 2019, and 2020, respectively, these models were visualized with improvements over the Ionic in terms of appearance that resembled the Apple Watch more closely. Fitbit Versa 2 integrated Amazon Alexa (the virtual assistant) for the first time, while Fitbit Versa 3 added GPS functionality and Google Assistant integration and a display with a higher resolution. Android users are also able to answer phone calls using Versa 3.
- *Fitbit Sense* – released in September 2020, has an echocardiogram (ECG) function and also has the capabilities for measuring blood oxygenation levels and stress tracking, which makes the Sense the most advanced product of the Fitbit brand.

Apart from fitness trackers and smartwatches, Fitbit also produces a smart scale. The first model was Fitbit Aria introduced in 2012 but was

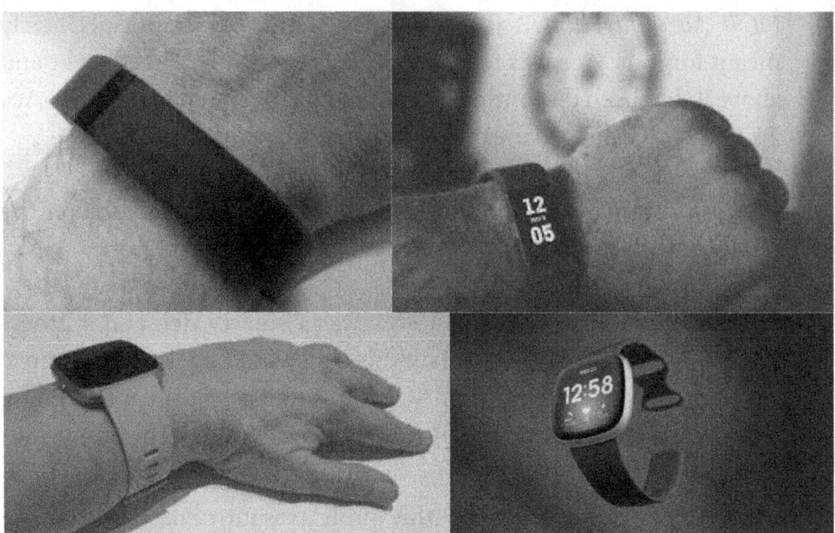

FIGURE 2.3 Some common Fitbit models – fitness trackers and smartwatches. (License: CC.)

replaced by the newer model Fitbit Aria 2 in August 2017. It is used to measure a user's body weight, BMI (body mass index), and percentage of body fat. It can track these body measurements and upload them onto the Fitbit app on a smartphone via Bluetooth capability. Aria 2 offers a more attractive and interactive design, better connectivity, and improved accuracy.

2.4.2 Apple Watch

Apple Watches are a line of smartwatches developed by Apple Inc., with the first model released in April 2015. It consists of an integrated technology for fitness tracking and other health-oriented functions and works primarily by pairing up with a compatible iPhone. Since its first appearance on the market, a new model has been introduced every year (typically in September) with new features and functions. Upon its release, it very quickly became a best-selling wearable device with millions of these being sold every year. Although exact sales figures for the Apple Watch are not known, it is estimated that by 2016, Apple had sold about 20 million watches and had a market share of 50%. We briefly summarize the different Apple Watch models below:

- *Apple Watch (first generation)* – first version released in 2015, but now discontinued

- *Apple Watch Series 1 and Series 2* – both released in 2016, these second models of the Apple Watch have also been discontinued now
- *Apple Watch Series 3* – this third version of the Apple Watch released in 2017 was equipped with LTE for the first time and hence was able to connect to a mobile network independently of an iPhone. This reduces its dependence on the phone, although the latter is required for the initial setup. This model is still available on the market.
- *Apple Watch Series 4* – released in 2018, this product has been discontinued.
- *Apple Watch Series 5* – released in 2019.
- *Apple Watch Series 6* – released in September 2020, this model introduced functionalities such as ECG and blood oxygenation level measurements for the Apple Watch line.
- *Apple Watch Series SE* – released in September 2020, this is a more affordable version of Apple Watch Series 6.
- *Apple Watch Series 7* – released in September 2021, this is by far the most advanced Apple Watch in terms of health indicators and is the most recent model currently available in the market. Apart from similar health innovations as the Apple Watch series 6, it also comes equipped with sleep tracking and mindfulness tracking.

Several modern designs, including a sport version and one with a stainless-steel body, are available today for the Apple Watch, thus making the product extremely attractive to a wide range of consumers in different markets. Apple Watch runs *watchOS*, whose interface consists of a home screen with circular app icons. Navigation is possible via the

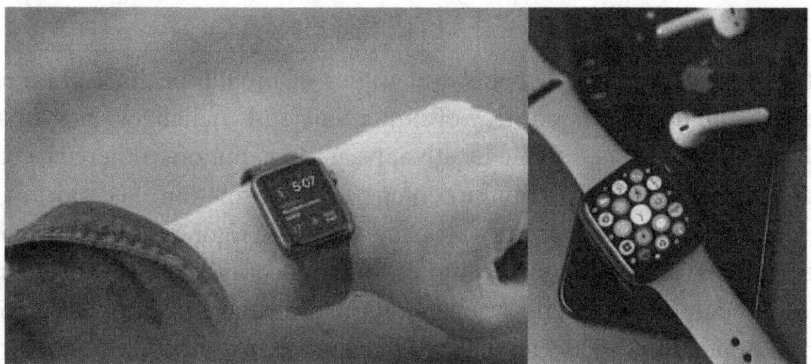

FIGURE 2.4 Apple Watch. (License: CC.)

touchscreen of the watch face, and it is typically paired with an iPhone to install updates, install new apps from the App Store, and customize other settings.

The Apple Watch can help users to track their physical activity in terms of the number of steps taken, active minutes, calories burned, pace, and distance covered (in mileage terms). It can track these activity metrics when a user is walking, running, swimming, hiking, rowing, or when exercising. WatchOS 3, released in 2016, introduced heart-rate monitoring and the 'Breathe' app, which encourages users to set aside a few minutes every day to relax and focus on breathing. The device is capable of receiving notifications, text messages, and phone calls via a paired mobile device. WatchOS5 introduced 'social networking' functionalities in the watch, thus encouraging users to connect with friends and family to share activity progress and participate in challenges and competition. Very recently, the Apple Watch Series 4 supports an integrated feature that can perform an electrocardiogram (also known as an ECG and EKG) via electrodes attached to the back of the watch's digital crown. It informs a user as to whether his/her heart has a normal rhythm or is experiencing any abnormal patterns, but it does not help diagnose any heart disease such as a heart attack. Another useful feature available on the Apple Watch Series 4, especially for older people, is fall detection. If a fall is detected, it sounds an alarm and provides the user with an option to tap it as a way to let it know that he/she is ok. If there is no timely response, the watch automatically calls emergency services for help. One potential drawback of the Apple Watch is that it is not able to track sleep and monitor sleep patterns, mainly owing to the short battery life (often only 24 hours). However, it is possible to do so using some third-party apps available on the App Store, although it is not known specifically how accurate these are.

2.5 THE FUTURE OF MHEALTH TECHNOLOGY

Although the potential benefits and values of mobile health technology are vast, the domain is not free of limitations and challenges. First of all, although many of the mobile health apps are free, but often there is a cost associated with more premium content and information. Second, many of these applications currently lack the scientific rigor required to make them reliable and viable medical tools. Rapid technological advancements often predate governmental regulations. Unfortunately, clinical practice recommendations regarding the use of technology lag even further behind. This raises some urgent questions about the safety of popular mobile devices. It also suggests the need for careful monitoring of new digital inventions to assess their practical value, reliability, and suitability. As mobile health increases its presence in the healthcare arena, we need to be aware of false promises. This includes recognizing some of the limitations of modern technology. There are some apps that are not compatible with all the mobile operating systems. For instance, apps that are specifically developed for Apple iOS devices (iPad, iPhone) may not work as smoothly or have all the functionalities when used on the Android system.

Mobile applications have great potential, yet there is still plenty of room for improvement to fully maximize their potential benefit. With the increasing use of digital health apps, it has become essential to improve the design processes, so applications can be easy to use while still having the desired effect on the user. Despite this, the number of mHealth apps in the Apple Store keeps increasing, with tracking tools being the most popular among consumers, followed by medical resources, informational, and educational tools.

Considering wearable fitness trackers and smartwatches (with in-built activity trackers), these have come a long way from the simple pedometers to the ones with advanced features like receiving texts and emails, monitoring heart rates and ECGs, and social networking. Tracking health has thus become increasingly more engaging and effective. As mHealth continues to evolve to address critical issues in healthcare today, fitness trackers have also evolved from mere technology fads to being essential components of a healthy lifestyle for many individuals. However, some people argue that wearable technology has more or less reached its peak, given all the super advanced features available in most of them today, with very little scope for further enhancements. There is also not much significant difference in terms of functionalities (and sometimes even appearance) among the different models produced by the top vendors, hence causing sales to plummet in the last two to three years. In 2017, Fitbit sales dropped 35% for the first time in the first nine months. So, although we are seeing newer products in the market on a regular basis still at this time, much of the focus has shifted to a slightly different item – namely, clothing. Sensors are expected to be embedded in clothing and shoes that will be able to track physical activities and health conditions, and these will be referred to as 'smart clothing' or '*everydayables*.' IDC Mobile Device Trackers predict major growth in smart clothing over the next few years; their data estimates it will account for 9.4% of the share of wearables in the near future with 22.3 million garments shipped by then [16].

Mobile health technology also faces some of the same issues of privacy and data ownership as other digital health innovation. More transparency regarding the use of the data collected via the apps and user feedback are key components in ensuring that these applications are adopted widely and their benefits fully realized by the general population. In emerging medical models, patients' interests should be considered a top priority. We are continuing to become more engaged partners in our own healthcare, and mobile health is providing the needed tools to ensure this trend continues.

NOTES

1 https://qxmd.com/read-by-qxmd
2 www.medpagetoday.com/
3 https://appointik.in/
4 www.kareo.com/
5 www.noom.com
6 These are the release dates for the first model of each company's product in a specific category (standalone tracker, smartwatch, etc.).
7 All models that came out after this chapter was written are not included in this table.
8 All models that came out after this chapter was written are not included in this table.

REFERENCES

1. U.S. Food and Drug Administration (FDA) website. Link: www.fda.gov/medical-devices/digital-health/device-software-functions-including-mobile-medical-applications. Retrieved on December 10, 2019.
2. Research 2 Guidance. 325,000 mobile health apps available in 2017 – Android now the leading mHealth platform. Link: https://research2guidance.com/325000-mobile-health-apps-available-in-2017/. Retrieved on March 30, 2019.
3. Zion Market Research (2019). mHealth Apps market by type: Global industry perspective, comprehensive analysis, and forecast, 2018 – 2025. Published by Globe Newswire on January 24, 2019. Link: www.globenewswire.com/news-release/2019/01/24/1704860/0/en/Global-mHealth-Apps-Market-Will-Reach-USD-111-1-Billion-By-2025-Zion-Market-Research.html. Retrieved on March 31, 2019.
4. Islam, Z. (2012). Smartphones heavily decrease sales of iPod, MP3 players, Tom's Hardware. Link: www.tomshardware.com/news/Smartphones-iPod-MP3-Players-Sales,20062.html, published on December 30, 2012. Retrieved on November 10, 2021.

5. Dicianno, B. E., Parmanto, B., Fairman, A. D., Crytzer, T. M., Yu, D. X., Pramana, GzmHealth) technologies and application to rehabilitation. *Physical therapy*, *95*(3), 397–405. DOI: https://doi.org/10.2522/ptj.20130534
6. Mikulic, M. (2020). Apple App Store: number of available medical apps as of Q1 2020. Statista. Link: www.statista.com/statistics/779910/health-apps-available-ios-worldwide/. Published on May 13, 2020. Retrieved on August 11, 2020.
7. Mikulic, M. (2020). Google Play: number of available medical apps as of Q4 2020. Statista. Link: www.statista.com/statistics/779919/health-apps-available-google-play-worldwide/. Published on May 13, 2020. Retrieved on August 11, 2020.
8. Liquid State (2018). The Rise of mHealth Apps: A Market Snapshot. Link: https://liquid-state.com/mhealth-apps-market-snapshot/. Published on March 26, 2018. Retrieved on August 11, 2020.
9. Pew Research Report (2021).Mobile Fact Sheet. Link: www.pewresearch.org/internet/fact-sheet/mobile/, published on April 7, 2021. Retrieved on November 10, 2021.
10. mHealth Economics 2017. Current Status and Future Trends in Mobile Health. Link: https://research2guidance.com/product/mhealth-economics-2017-current-status-and-future-trends-in-mobile-health/. Published in November 2017. Retrieved on August 11, 2020.
11. Social Factor Blog (2021). Social Health Apps are the future of Personal Wellness. Link: https://socialfactor.com/blog/social-health-apps-impacting-personal-wellness/. Retrieved on August 21, 2021.
12. Douglas-Walton, J. (2021). A Study of fitness trackers and wearables. Link: www.hfe.co.uk/blog/a-study-of-fitness-trackers-and-wearables/, retrieved on November 20, 2021.
13. Pebble (Watch). Wikipedia page: https://en.wikipedia.org/wiki/Pebble_(watch).
14. McGuire, J. (2021). Best fitness trackers in 2021: Top activity bands from Fitbit, Garmin and more, *Tom's guide*, Link: www.tomsguide.com/us/best-fitness-trackers,review-2066.html, published on November 30, 2021. Retrieved on November 30, 2021.
15. Vailshery, L.S. (2020). Market share of wearables unit shipments worldwide from 2014 to 2020, by vendor. *Statista.com* Link: www.statista.com/statistics/515640/quarterly-wearables-shipments-worldwide-market-share-by-vendor/, published on September 7, 2021. Retrieved on November 20, 2021.
16. Fitt Insider (2020).The Rise, Fall, and Future of Wearable Fitness Devices. Link: https://insider.fitt.co/future-wearable-fitness/. Retrieved on August 17, 2020.

Appendix

TABLE 2A.1 Different models and versions of some of the well-known standalone fitness trackers and smartwatches produced by the top vendors today

Vendor	Fitness trackers (standalone)
Fitbit	Flex*, Flex 2*, Force*, Charge*, Charge 2*, Charge HR*, Alta*, Alta HR*, Ace, Charge 3, Charge 4, Inspire*, Inspire HR*, Inspire 2, Luxe, Charge 5
Jawbone	UP, UP24, UP2, Up3, UP4, Small UP
Nike	Fuelband*, Fuelband 2
Xiaomi	Mi Band, Mi Band 1S, Mi Band 2, Mi Band HRX Edition, Mi Band 3, Mi Band 4, Mi Band 5, Mi Band 6
Garmin	Vivosmart 3, Vivosmart 4, Vivosport
Samsung	Galaxy Fit, Fit 2 Pro, Gear Fit 2
Huawei	Fit, Band 3, Band 2, Band 2 pro, Band 3 Pro, Band, Band 4, Band 4 Pro, Honor Band 5, Honor Band 4, Honor Band 3, Honor Band 2, Honor Band
TomTom	Cardio

Most well-known manufacturers of fitness trackers (standalone) and selected models for each[7]. * denotes a discontinued model.

Vendor	Smartwatches
Fitbit	Surge*, Blaze*, Ionic*, Versa, Versa 2, Versa Lite, Versa 3, Sense
Apple	Apple Watch Series 7, Watch Series 6, Watch SE, Watch Series 5, Watch Series 4, Watch Series 3, Watch Series 2, Watch Series 1
Apple + Nike	Apple Watch Nike Series 5, Apple Watch Nike
Xiaomi	Mi Watch, Amazfit, Redmi Band, Amazfit Verge, Amazfit Pace, Amazfit GTR
Garmin	Fenix 6, Forerunner 45, Forerunner 945, Vivoactive 4, Vivoactive 3, Vivoactive 2, Vivoactive, Vivoactive HR, Venu 2, Lily
Samsung	Galaxy Watch 3, Galaxy Watch 2, Galaxy Watch, Galaxy Watch Active 2, Galaxy Watch Active, Gear Sport, Galaxy Gear, Gear S, Gear 2, Gear 2 Neo, Gear Live
Huawei	Watch GT 2, Watch GT, Watch GT Sport, Watch GT 2e, Watch GT Active Edition, Watch GT Elegant Edition, Watch 2 Sport, Watch 3
Verizon	Gizmo Watch, Wear24, Motorola Moto 360 Sports
Asus	Vivowatch, Vivowatch SP
Withings	Steel HR, Steel HR Sport, Move ECG, Withings Move
Timex	iConnect, iConnect Active, iConnect Pro, iConnect Premium Active, Metropolitan, Ironman

Most well-known manufacturers of fitness trackers and smartwatches and selected models for each[8]. * denotes a discontinued model.

CHAPTER 3

How Does mHealth Technology Work?

3.1 INTRODUCTION

mHealth technology has pervaded the markets today. They have evolved from just being technology fads to becoming essential and critical to ensuring health and wellness of a large population of consumers today. People have realized the potential health benefits offered by this technology and hence have been open to embracing it for their own health management. However, it is important to understand how these trackers work, how they collect and track data over time, and how consumers can read that data and understand and interpret them in a way that will be beneficial to their overall health.

In this chapter, we discuss in details how different kinds of mHealth technology work, starting with mobile health applications (apps), followed by the wearable devices. With the explosive growth of all aspects of technology over the past decade and a half, this domain has been seeded, grown, and flourished in the United States and across the world, so much so that we can now have important health-related data at our fingertips (literally) anytime anywhere. mHealth is considered as a subset of 'telehealth' (or 'telemedicine'), which was introduced decades ago to extend the reach of healthcare beyond traditional medical settings via electronic and telecommunication tools, by leveraging the growth and development of digital technology. This type of sustained monitoring helps diagnose a disease or detect a potentially dangerous health condition early on so that suitable

DOI: 10.1201/9780429428449-3

treatment and intervention can be implemented as quickly as possible. For example, an irregular heart rate or high blood pressure measured by a fitness tracker can indicate a heart condition and, in some cases, even an imminent heart attack. Early detection can lead to timely consultation with a physician and hence the appropriate steps to address this issue. This is where the power and strength of mobile health technology lie today.

This chapter is organized as follows. Section 3 2 presents a description of how mobile health apps work, and Section 3.3 discusses how different wearable fitness trackers work with a focus on a few common ones. Section 3.4 presents some issues and challenges associated with mHealth technology, and we conclude with a brief discussion and conclusion in Section 3.5.

3.2 MOBILE HEALTH APPS

Mobile health applications (or apps) are applications that function on mobile devices, such as smartphones, personal digital assistants, and tablet computers. A wide range of mobile health applications are now available today on most mainstream mobile platforms, such as Apple and Samsung. According to a report published by Statista Research Department, Google Play was the app store with the largest number of mobile health apps at 3.48 million, followed by 2.22 million such apps available on the Apple App Store at the end of March 2021 ([1]).

As with any mobile app, these apps can be pre-installed on mobile devices through manufacturers (such as *Samsung Health* on Samsung Galaxy phones or *iHealth* app on iPhones) or purchased and installed by users after they buy a device through the manufacturer's app store (for example, the Apple Store for iPhone or iPad users or Google Play Store for Android-based phone users), or even delivered as web applications that could be accessed through a regular web browser on any computer or mobile device. These applications are also required to be optimized for different operating systems of the mobile devices, as they are very different (like Android and iOS), for different hardware specifications and configurations (like screen sizes) and compatibility with different internal functions. The apps have software programs embedded within them that enable the collection of different types of health, fitness, and medical data. Once the data are obtained, they are stored, processed, and converted into meaningful output to be shared with the users or medical professionals based on the need and purposed of the app. Lastly, as discussed in the next section, almost all of the wearable fitness trackers have mobile apps that are installed on a mobile phone that has to be paired or synced with the device and are able to display fitness and health data once they are collected, compiled, and analyzed. All the different types of mobile health apps available in the market today are described in detail in Chapter 2.

Given the popularity of Samsung smartphones today, **Samsung Health** is a mobile health app used today by many. It is equipped with several features and can track one's weight (needs to be entered by the user), calorie intake, calories burnt, number of steps, heart rate, stress levels, caffeine intake, water intake, blood pressure, sleep, and so on. Sometimes the large number of features and measurements can be overwhelming and confusing, so users have the option to pick and choose what works for them using the 'manage items' button displayed at the bottom of the app. Figure 3.1 below shows a typical dashboard of Samsung Health as seen on a Samsung phone.

Many mobile health apps also came into existence and quickly became popular during the COVID-19 pandemic that started since March 2020. One such app is called **Othena**,[1] created for providing vaccination guidelines and information to Orange County (California) residents in early 2021. It is built as a 'SaaS' platform (Software as a Service) so that people can download and install it as an application on their mobile devices. It offers an easy way of registering for vaccination, scheduling appointments, and obtaining notifications when a vaccine becomes available in the user's area via emails and text messages. Othena also provides updated data about vaccine requirements, testing locations, availability, distribution, and shipment tracking, along with useful resources about up-to-date CDC guidelines

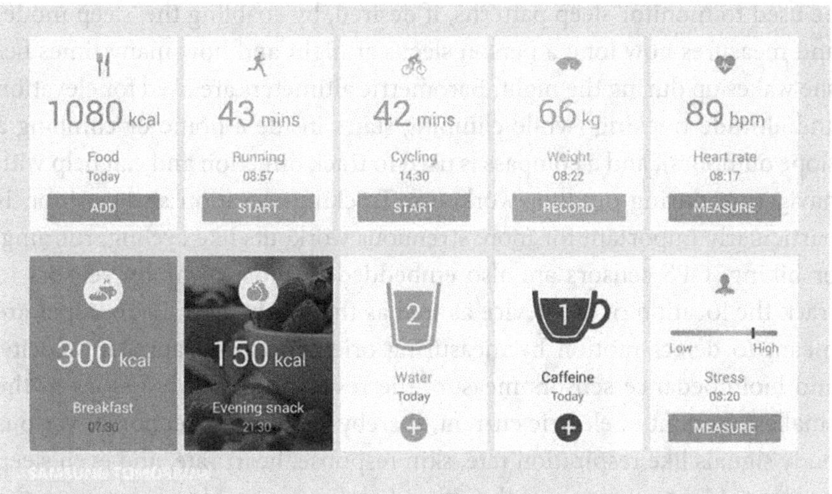

FIGURE 3.1 Samsung Health app dashboard. (License: CC.)

about the coronavirus and other public health services in the county. As of September 20, 2021, this app had 1,371,295 patients registered and reported having administered 1,241,997 doses of vaccine to date.

3.3 WEARABLE FITNESS TRACKERS

Wearable fitness trackers typically consist of a mini-computer that uses sensors to gather different types of data about a person's activity and body ([2]). Some common types of sensors integrated with fitness trackers are as follows:

- Accelerometers and motion sensors
- Altimeters
- Compass
- GPS
- Gyroscopes
- Bioimpedance sensors
- Ambient light sensors
- Proximity sensors

Accelerometers are used to detect and track movement (count the number of steps, physical activity, speed, calories burnt) and acceleration, while motion sensors track different types of physical activities, such as running, jogging, cycling, swimming, and walking. These sensors also can be used to monitor sleep patterns, if desired, by enabling the 'sleep mode,' and measures how long a person sleeps at night and how many times he/she wakes up during the night. Barometric altimeters are used for elevation and altitude tracking (while climbing stairs inside a home or climbing a slope outdoors), and a compass is used to track direction and can help with navigation during outdoor workouts. Tracking elevation and position is particularly important for more strenuous workouts like cycling, running, or hiking. GPS sensors are also embedded in most common sensors to track the location of the device as well as that of the user. Gyroscopes are meant to detect motion by measuring orientation and angular velocity, and bioimpedance sensors measure the resistance of body tissues to the smallest amount of electric current, thereby enabling collection of various body signals like respiration rate, skin response, heart rate, and even sleep patterns. Light sensors, on the other hand, are capable of detecting the amount of light in the surrounding areas and adjust the display brightness accordingly. Proximity sensors help a tracking device to conserve battery by sleeping when not in use and wake up the display as soon as the user is near the device and wants to use it.

With time, fitness trackers have evolved, and current ones come equipped with a lot of additional sensors for measuring and monitoring a variety of activities and health indicators. Some of these are enumerated below, along with their specific functionalities:

- Optical heart rate sensor for detecting heart beats per minute – the sensor shines a light through the skin to detect blood flow and measure how many times the heart beats per minute
- SpO2 sensor to measure blood oxygen levels
- ECG sensors to detect and measure the electrical impulse sent out by each heartbeat (as in an echocardiogram) – this sensor detects this minute heart signal through the electrodes embedded in the wearable device
- Gesture sensors to detect wrist motion
- UV sensors to measure exposure to harmful sunlight
- Magnetometer, used in conjunction with the GPS and compass, to determine the exact coordinates of a user's location
- Electrodermal activity sensor to measure stress, along with a heart rate tracker and ECG by detecting small electrical changes in the sweat level of the skin
- Skin temperature sensor to monitor slight changes in temperature to determine whether the user is going to get a fever and fall sick and also to detect the start of a menstrual cycle in women

Many of these sensors can be used together; for example, one of Garmin's devices combines the altimeter, barometer, and compass with GPS and gives more precise details on movements. In other instances, these sensors can function alone to yield individual measurements as desired by the user. Once the readings are recorded, the data are stored and processed by the underlying software algorithms integrated with the device to translate them into helpful and user-friendly figures, such as mileage covered during a run or the number of 'very active minutes' of physical activity or health readings like pulse rate and blood oxygen levels.

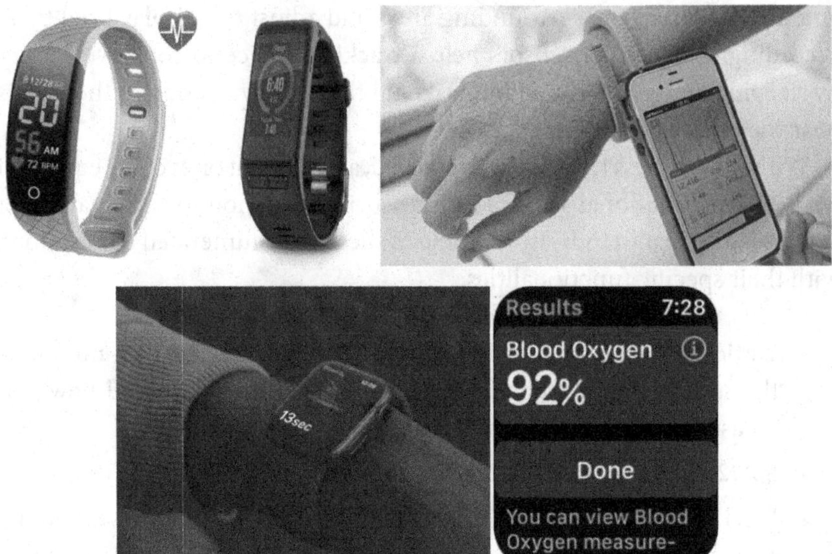

FIGURE 3.2 Some common measurements recorded by wearable fitness trackers like heart rate, sleep, blood oxygen levels, and physical activity. (License: CC.)

Today, many tools are available that enable most wearable fitness devices to be synced or paired with an app on smartphones and/or tablet computers. For example, *Fitbit SDK*[2] allows the development of the Fitbit app for mobile devices and clock face for various Fitbit models, and Fitbit API is used by developers to access Fitbit activity data from users; *WatchKit*[3] is the developer toolkit for Apple Watch models to sync with iPhones; and *Wear OS*[4] is a version of Google's Android operating system for smartwatches and other wearable devices. Similarly, Garmin had its own tools for creating applications for Garmin devices.[5] These apps help users visualize and analyze their activity levels and habits via 'data dashboards' – a collection of charts, graphs, and data tables created based on the collected measurements. Moreover, one can share these results with others via a leaderboard that tap into social networking capabilities ([3]).

Fitness trackers thus help individuals monitor and keep track of their own health by letting them set health goals, set reminders for activities such as drinking water frequently and meeting daily exercise and dietary needs. All of these not only help them maintain a healthy lifestyle but also make positive changes to further improve their health. Additionally, the ability to track others' fitness goals and share one's own progress motivates people to stay on track and meet their fitness targets. Massive amounts of data are available at the fingertips of users who have developed a sense of community among those with similar fitness and health goals. Using these trackers, an individual can thus limit the number of calorie intake, focus on sleeping and eating habits, and strive to achieve daily exercise targets, along with motivating others to do the same. In March 2020, the COVID-19 pandemic started raging worldwide; it limited people's movements outdoors, and closed gyms and training facilities, thus making it difficult for people to maintain their exercise and fitness regimes. In such a scenario, fitness trackers had the potential to encourage people to keep exercising and stay active while being connected and communicating with other people at the same time.

3.3.1 Common Wearable Fitness Trackers

Fitbit Versa, the Charge and Inspire series, Garmin Forerunner, the Apple Watch series, and the Samsung watch series are among the most popular fitness trackers in the market. Depending on the budget and features desired, users, however, may prefer a variety of other brands that have emerged in this field.

Taking a deeper look at **Fitbit Charge 4**, the latest Fitbit model released in 2020, we see that it consists of a three-axis accelerometer to track motion patterns; an optical heart-rate monitor; a GPS receiver to track location during workouts; infrared sensors to detect SpO2 oxygen saturation levels; a temperature sensor for the skin; a vibration motor for haptics like alarm, notifications, reminders, and apps; wireless technology using an NFC chip and altimeter to track altitude changes; and a rechargeable lithium-polymer battery. Fitbit Charge 4 also monitors stress levels and sleep patterns and keeps track of women's menstrual cycles. An optical heart-rate sensor flashes green LEDs multiple times in a second and makes use of light-sensitive photodiodes to detect blood volume changes in the capillaries above the wrist. Then the device computes the number of heartbeats per minute (bpm). Some additional features on this device include the capability to listen to music via Spotify (subscription needed), make contactless payments from the wrist without a wallet using Fitbit Pay,[6] and receive notifications about calls, texts, and meeting reminders from a paired smartphone (replies to texts can be made for an Android phone but not for an iPhone). A user can also enter their information such as age, weight, height, gender, etc., for a user profile. The algorithms embedded

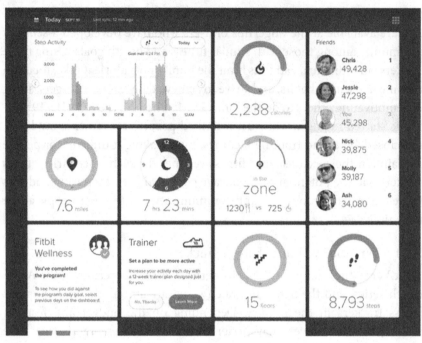

FIGURE 3.3 A typical dashboard for Fitbit Charge 4, as shown on the Fitbit mobile app. (License: CC.)

in the tracker can then use these data to calculate the health metrics for display and visualizations in the form of graphs to determine trends and patterns. Figure 3.3 below shows a typical dashboard for Fitbit Charge 4.

Among smartwatches, the most popular models are the Apple Watches. **Apple Watch Series 6**, the latest line of models released in 2020, introduced a blood oxygen sensor and an ECG sensor for the first time in Apple Watch history. Electrodes are embedded in the watch, which can read a heart's electrical signals to determine if the heart is beating in a normal sinus rhythm or to detect any abnormal heart rhythm that can signal signs of atrial fibrillation. The blood oxygen sensor, on the other hand, has four LED clusters and four photodiodes to determine one's blood oxygen level. Green and red LED lights are shone on the wrist, and the amount of light reflected is measured by the photodiodes that are used by advanced algorithms to determine the color of the blood and hence the oxygenation level of the blood (bright red blood is oxygenated, while dark red blood denotes a lower amount of oxygen). Other regular features include accelerometers, altimeters, GPS, compasses, etc., for tracking movement and physical

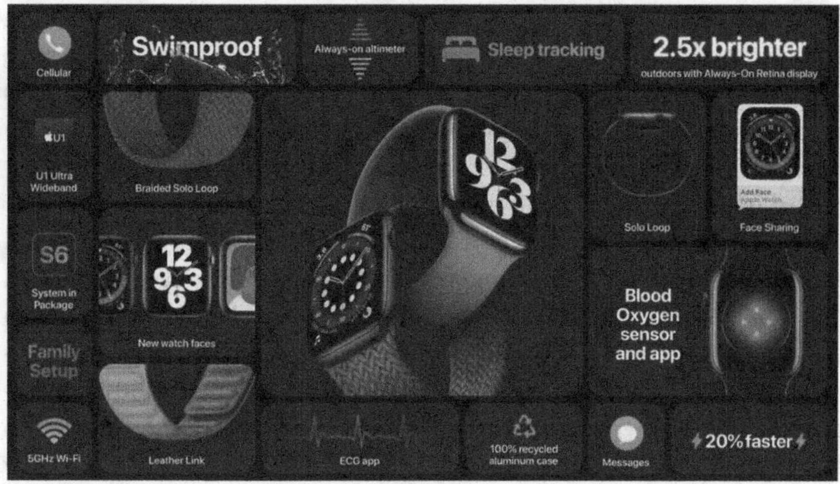

FIGURE 3.4 A snapshot of the mobile app dashboard for Apple Watch Series 6. (License: CC.)

activity levels, a gyroscope, a heart-rate monitor, a sleep monitor, and an ambient light sensor. All of these activity and health readings can be monitored and observed by the user on the watch face itself or on the watch app on a paired iPhone. Moreover, just like Fitbits, Apple Watches also come equipped with Apple Pay, a contactless payment method that stores a user's credit and debit card information digitally, and it works from the watch itself or from the mobile app. Finally, the watch is water-resistant and therefore can be worn during swimming, diving, and other water sports and activities, can be used to listen to music, and can receive and answer phone calls and texts received through the paired iPhone. Figure 3.4 shows a snapshot of all the functionalities of an Apple Watch (Series 6) as it shows on the mobile app.

3.4 ISSUES AND CHALLENGES WITH MHEALTH FUNCTIONALITIES

The use of fitness trackers or mHealth apps has been seen as a trend in the past few years, but these days, they have evolved as a need. Despite the tremendous growth of fitness trackers (wearables as well as apps), there are certain concerns among users pertaining to the use of these devices/apps. One of the main concerns revolves around security/data privacy. The messages or data transmission between trackers and servers could be hacked and could pose potential risk to users' personal information and health data that are of extremely sensitive nature. Even the systems with encryption could be affected by security issues. Along with the issues surrounding the trackers, some individuals share their tracker data on social media, which further adds to the security concerns. These privacy-related issues are discussed in more detail in Chapter 6.

Another concern regarding mHealth technology is the reliability and accuracy of the data collected and reported. Some reports have mentioned that popular devices like Fitbit often underestimate and overestimate step count data in some situations [4]. Other devices have been known to estimate health readings only approximately, such as heart rate and temperature [5]. In some cases, playing the piano or cooking has been seen to add to the step count on a wearable device, although the person is only moving his/her hands while remaining stationary. The blood oxygen levels measured by Apple Watch (Series 6) can sometimes be misleading if a person has tattoos on the wrist, as tattoo ink can make it hard for the light from the LED sensors to reach the blood vessels under the skin. Moreover, the data need to be presented in a meaningful and user-friendly way that can be easily understood by the consumer that can also motivate further action in terms of lifestyle changes if needed. Some other factors, particularly for wearable devices, like short battery life (for example, some Apple Watches need to be charged everyday), ease and convenience of use, and the price of the device can adversely affect a person's motivation and desire to use them on a continuous basis.

3.5 CONCLUSIONS

The world has seen a wide range of products on fitness tracking in the last decade or so. Some are easier to use, and some are more budget friendly, while others vary on features. The growing use of trackers among people has led to innovations in this field, leading to fancier and trendier new designs and looks. The COVID-19 pandemic has also made people more aware of the need to stay active and healthy on their own, which has also impacted a more widespread adoption and use of mHealth technology (both wearable devices and mobile apps). Apple's market share for Apple Watch has increased significantly in the recent months, and it emerged as a market leader in mobile health in 2021 [6]. In particular, the integration of health indicators such as blood pressure, heart rate, and blood oxygen levels, among others, in the most modern trackers (like the Apple Watch) have yielded individuals with an easy and quick way at their fingertips to monitor their health in a regular way without having to visit a doctor's office. This has reduced crowds at hospitals and clinics, brought down healthcare costs and insurance premiums (as diseases can be diagnosed and remedied much more quickly), and made people more productive at work, as they do not need to take time off any more in the middle of a workday to keep doctors' appointments. Similarly, if people do not have time to go a gym to get their daily exercise, they can still work out at home (or at work, depending on the situation) and monitor their physical activity with the help of fitness trackers. In this way, they can remain active and healthy without having to travel to another location that saves time and other resources (like car fuel) too.

However, as more and more data are being collected with more usage, privacy and security concerns have also grown, with increasing incidents of data breaches and leaks. Companies are working to overcome these challenges as quickly as possible to assure their consumers and restore their confidence in the products, along with the government, which is working in some sectors to set guidelines for the developers as well as users to prevent such data losses in the future. Manufacturers of fitness trackers and mobile health apps also need to conduct more research into the accuracy and reliability of measurements collected by these devices and make the necessary adjustments and improvements to their software algorithms based on that. This can potentially further increase the market for these devices and applications and lead to greater overall health for the population at large.

NOTES

1 www.othena.com/
2 https://dev.fitbit.com/
3 https://developer.apple.com/documentation/watchkit
4 https://wearos.google.com/#hands-free-help
5 https://developer.garmin.com/
6 www.fitbit.com/global/us/technology/fitbit-pay

REFERENCES

1. Statista Research Department (2021). Link: www.statista.com/statistics/276623/number-of-apps-available-in-leading-app-stores/. Published on September 10, 2021, retrieved on September 20, 2021.

2. Roberts, A. (2019). The Best Fitness Trackers, WireCutter review, link: https://thewirecutter.com/reviews/the-best-fitness-trackers/, published on February 8, 2019. Retrieved on February 25, 2019.
3. CNN Report (2013). Fitness tools that ta the power of your friends. Link: www.cnn.com/2013/06/03/tech/mobile/fitness-gadgets-motivation/–Fitness Studies get Social, published on June 3, 2013. Retrieved March 26, 2015.
4. Feehan, L. M., Geldman, J., Sayre, E. C., Park, C., Ezzat, A. M., Yoo, J. Y., Hamilton, C. B., & Li, L. C. (2018). Accuracy of Fitbit Devices: Systematic Review and Narrative Syntheses of Quantitative Data, *Journal of Medical Internet Research* (JMIR); mHealth and uHealth, 6(8), e10527. Doi: https://doi.org/10.2196/10527
5. Kroll, R.R., Boyd, J.G., Maslove, D.M. (2016). Accuracy of a Wrist-Worn Wearable Device for Monitoring Heart Rates in Hospital Inpatients: A Prospective Observational Study, *Journal of Medical Internet Research* (JMIR); 18(9), e 253. doi2196/jmir.6025
6. Vailshery, L.S. (2021). Market share of wearables unit shipments worldwide from 1Q'14 to 1Q'21, by vendor. Link: www.statista.com/statistics/435944/quarterly-wearables-shipments-worldwide-market-share-by-vendor/. Retrieved on August 30, 2021.

CHAPTER 4

Advances in mHealth Research

4.1 INTRODUCTION

As wearable technology in the form of electronic fitness tracking devices and smartwatches become a more and more popular means of encouraging physical activity and impacting health behaviors, a natural question that arises is that whether these devices are actually able to help consumers achieve their health goals and maintain a healthy lifestyle. Towards this, much research has been conducted in the past few years on the efficacy, accuracy, utility, and reliability of mobile health devices. The purpose of research is to inform society about emerging technologies and their impact, thus advancing knowledge and driving decisions and actions. It provides consumers with the necessary data and results or findings to understand their functionalities and potential benefits, which in turn drives decisions regarding whether to adopt such tracking devices for their own personal health management. To date, research on mobile healthcare has been based on both randomized controlled trials and observation studies. Several meta-analytic studies have also been conducted to assess the different types of health impacts of mobile health technology on a larger scale.

This chapter provides a summary of selected existing research on different aspects of mobile health or fitness trackers and is organized as follows. Section 4.2 presents an overview of research on the impact of electronic fitness tracking devices on personal health; Section 4.3 discusses research on the utility, accuracy, and reliability of the measurements

DOI: 10.1201/9780429428449-4

captured by these trackers; and Section 4.4 presents existing works on the security of data collected these devices. Finally, Section 4.5 concludes with an overview of challenges that researchers encounter in this area, along with potential future research directions.

4.2 IMPACT ON PERSONAL HEALTH

Although nearly half of U.S. adults are overweight or obese, according to the Centers for Disease Control and Prevention (www.cdc.gov/obesity/data/adult.html), only 45% of Americans get enough physical activity, which creates a significant public health concern. Physical activity is associated with improvement in many health conditions: obesity; reducing the risk of cardiovascular disease, type 2 diabetes, and metabolic syndrome; some cancers; and mental health disorders. Guidelines from the Department of Health and Human Services (www.hhs.gov) recommend that adults get at least 30 minutes of daily physical activity, and several organizations and medical professionals recommend that adults walk 10,000 steps each day. We categorize the studies below based on the type of mobile health technology used - pedometers, wearable trackers, mobile health apps, and wearable trackers + mobile apps.

4.2.1 Pedometers

One of the earliest studies on fitness trackers involved pedometers, which are small, inexpensive devices designed to count the number of steps a person takes in a day. These are easy to use and can be clipped to the user's pocket or waistline. Researchers at Stanford University discovered that pedometer use helped improve blood pressure and increased physical activity and weight loss [1]. In fact, these devices were found to increase physical activity by 2,000 daily steps, or about 1 mile of walking. [2] presented an overview of existing research on the impact of pedometers on chronic conditions in adults that included type 2 diabetes, arthritis, hypertension, heart disease, or obesity. Their results suggested a potential benefit of pedometer use interventions for older adults for weight loss, although the average amount of weight loss attained was quite small. Similarly, increases in levels of physical activity were also observed in adults with other chronic conditions like type 2 diabetes and hypertension.

Focusing on young adults, a study based on 113 junior high school students (seventh and eighth graders) did not find statistically significant differences in the levels of physical activities among pedometer users and non-users, although some self-regulation strategies such as having access to and charting daily step counts positively influenced young adolescents to attain a higher number of daily steps [3]. Cayir et al. conducted a randomized controlled trial in 2015 among obese women enrolled in a university in Turkey to assess the efficacy of a pedometer-based intervention to increase physical activity and impact weight loss [4]. Their experiments based on 84 women showed that not only was the level of physical activity significantly higher for the intervention group, but weight, body mass index (BMI), body fat percentage, and waist circumference measurements also significantly decreased for the pedometer-intervention group compared to the control group (p-value < 0.001).

4.2.2 Wearable Fitness Trackers

Although step counting is the main function of wearable fitness trackers, the tracking of heart rate, calories burned, distance traveled, and sleep quality are also increasingly being used by consumers. By adopting and using these fitness devices, people are thus able to not only monitor their physical activity but also monitor their health conditions on a daily basis. Hence, research on fitness trackers has expanded to several aspects of human health and well-being beyond physical activity.

One recent study [5] based on a longitudinal randomized controlled trial using a pre-post design found that wearing a self-tracking device had a statistically small but significant positive effect on users' perceived physical health and their sense of accomplishment compared to the control group, while health consciousness increased for all participants in the study. Another study [6] conducted among college students who were provided with fitness trackers to assess their impact did not indicate a significant change in number of daily steps over 12 weeks or in any of the body measurements, such as body composition, resting heart rate, and blood pressure. However, some positive outcomes were observed as well in terms of increase in knowledge and self-perception of wellness because of participation in this study.

A recent meta-analysis study [7] observed a significant increase in daily step count, moderate to high levels of physical activity, and a non-significant decrease in sedentary behavior for the group that underwent intervention in the form of a wearable activity tracker. [8] performed an observational study to explore whether fitness trackers increased the level of physical activity for older adults with multiple sclerosis (MS). Based on survey responses from 440 participants, only 28% used fitness trackers, with Fitbit, Apple Watch, and Garmin being the most popular ones. Further, strong correlations were observed with physical activity levels and fitness tracker usage that indicated the importance of this technology as a behavioral tool to increase levels of physical activity among the MS population, which usually has alarmingly low levels of such activities.

Fitness trackers are increasingly being used by different organizations (business and universities) as part of corporate wellness programs to promote and encourage healthier lifestyles among employees. There are many advantages to a healthy workforce, including increased productivity and lower health insurance premiums. Already nearly 2,000 companies worldwide offer fitness trackers to their employees, some examples being Target and Barclays [9,10]. Some of these companies even provide additional incentives to their employees for participating and sharing their information. A recent research study [11] examined the impact of providing a wearable fitness tracker as well as financial incentives on physical activity levels among employees at a public regional university. The findings showed that activity levels of employees increased with the incentives, although the reported improvement in health were low-moderate with only 4 to 18% of improvements in health attributable only to program participation. [12] proposed a case study at a financial institution in the southern United States that was providing Fitbits to their employees to motivate them to be healthier. The researchers administered surveys to both participants in the company's wellness programs and determine their usage patterns and motivation behind the use and to non-participants to learn about their reasons for abstaining from the program. The results suggested that extended use of Fitbit features had a positive impact on employee wellbeing and step count. A pilot study among employees at a healthcare facility who were at risk for chronic diseases (mostly women and in the overweight category) discovered that certain physiological indicators of health, such as blood pressure, waist measurements, etc., improved with the use of electronic fitness trackers and remote interaction and support from researchers [13].

Not all research studies on fitness trackers report positive outcomes. A randomized controlled trial involving 800 subjects conducted between June 2013 and August 2014 found that after one year of use, a fitness tracker had no effect on the subjects' overall health and fitness, despite the offer of financial incentives [14]. Another randomized controlled trial conducted by researchers at the University of Pittsburgh between October 2010 and October 2012 studied whether combining a fitness tracker with a weight loss program was effective in helping individual lose more weight and improve overall health [15]. Their results showed that subjects who did not use the fitness tracker lost more weight than those who did not use them, and the level of physical activity was also more or less the same for both groups.

4.2.3 Mobile Health (mHealth) Apps

Just as with wearable fitness trackers, mobile health (mHealth) apps have also been studied in the literature for their impact on personal health and wellness management as they become increasingly popular for medical interventions in different sectors of healthcare today.

[16] discussed how different mHealth apps have the potential of impacting patient health, particularly for the self-management of chronic diseases. An early literature search-based study [17] evaluated the efficacy of phone voice and text message-based interventions to address chronic diseases in adults in low- or middle-income countries. They discovered that there was overall improvement in clinical and chronic disease outcomes, attendance rates at clinics and hospitals, and general health-related quality of life for participants. [18] studied the influence of a mobile fitness application designed to enhance physical functioning of individuals via prescribed physical movements and exercises based on individual movement assessment. Based on a randomized controlled trial involving 48 healthy adults, they observed that the app improved indices of functional movement, flexibility (like shoulder and dorsiflexion), and muscular endurance over an eight-week period, whereas no changes were observed in handgrip strength, lower body power, and cardiovascular fitness between the experimental and control groups. Based on a large-scale randomized experiment designed in partnership with a major mHealth app platform, one study [19] observed that the adoption of the app not only improved people's health (such as reduction in blood glucose levels and glycated hemoglobin levels) but also significantly reduced patient hospital visits and associated medical expenses.

Based on a meta-analytic study of five electronic databases, [20] found that mHealth app interventions were associated with decreases in sedentary time, increases in physical activity time, and increases in overall fitness among a sample of older adults over a three-month period, although the statistical significance of the results could not be established. The authors thus suggested a larger study with longer follow-up periods in order to fully assess the value of mHealth apps in delivering sustained positive health outcomes. Similarly, [21] found that the impact of health interventions aimed at promoting health and disease management was weak based on systematic review and meta-analysis of randomized controlled trials. Another study [22] examined 23 mHealth apps prescribed by doctors to patients suffering from health conditions such as diabetes, mental health, and obesity. Their findings showed limited evidence of the impact of these apps on positive health outcomes for patients.

Recently, since the novel coronavirus driven pandemic started in early 2020, the use of mobile health apps and telemedicine has increased tremendously in applications, such as setting up virtual clinics, remote consultations with medical professionals like doctors and nurses, remote prescription fillings, and remote data sharing (like X-rays and scans) during the forced lockdown period [23]. Not only that, but coronavirus testing and vaccination processes were also mostly managed through mobile apps. A study of 29 apps showed that 15 (52%) were meant for contact tracing of COVID-19, 7 (24%) were meant for providing guidance on quarantine in the event of the exposure to the disease, 7 (24%) were meant for monitoring symptoms, and 1 (10%) was devised for disseminating information to the general population [24]. More recently [25] presented an overview of and taxonomy of all the different health apps available in the market to combat COVID-19 based on their purpose and features. Of the 115 apps that the study included, 77 (67%) were developed by governments and national authorities and were meant for users to monitor their own health for potential COVID-19 symptoms. Other app features included raising awareness about the disease and safety protocols to protect oneself from the disease, self-managing exposure to the disease, monitoring of health by doctors and other medical professionals, and conducting research studies.

4.2.4 Wearable Fitness Trackers and mHealth Apps

Several research works have focused on both wearable fitness trackers and mobile health apps. Based on a meta-analysis of 28 studies involving nearly 7,500 individuals, [26] showed that wearable fitness trackers as well as smartphone apps worked well in terms of increasing physical activity when they provided feedback on progress, enabled users to set personal goals, or reminded them to get active via text message notifications. In fact, people using these devices were found to walk an additional 1,850 steps daily. Wearable trackers included in the study were *Fitbit*, *Fitbug*,[1] *Withings Activite Steel*,[2] and *Jawbone*, and a variety of smartphone apps were included, like *Moves* and *Accupedo-Pro*.

4.3 RESEARCH ON ACCURACY, RELIABILITY, USABILITY, AND UTILITY OF MHEALTH TECHNOLOGY

Several studies have focused on establishing the reliability of fitness trackers and comparing accuracy of the different fitness trackers currently available on the market. For example, Caitlin et al. (2015) compared five different popular trackers: Nike + Fuelband, Fitbit Ulta, Jawbone UP, BodyMedica FitCore, and the Adidas MiCoach in terms of their accuracy in tracking steps and calories expended in several different types of physical activities, such as treadmill walking, elliptical use, treadmill running, and so on. Similarly, other studies [27] have determined that some measurements (like step counts) may be more or less accurate and lie within 9% of the actual steps, whereas others (like distance traveled) may not be so. One study found that the faster the walking speed, the greater is the error for the distance measure for pedometers, especially when kept in a pocket or in a purse [28] and suggests that they should be placed at the waist or in the arm for more accurate measurements. A more recent study with 24 participants found that Fitbit Blaze device's accelerometer and pulse data were not as accurate as those from medical grade devices [29]. A systematic review of literature presented by [30] showed that Fitbit devices accurately report step counts approximately half of the time, with overestimation occurring mostly in real-life settings and underestimation in controlled settings. Moreover, metrics such as calories burned are also often not accurately measured by such devices. An observational study conducted in a real-life setting [31] demonstrated that heart rates monitored by wearable fitness trackers were slightly lower than those derived for ECG monitoring and recommended further studies to evaluate such accuracies in order for fitness trackers to be more widely deployed in hospitals and clinical settings as early warning systems for cardiovascular diseases.

[32] conducted an observational study to assess the utility of wearable fitness trackers. A total of 47 participants (mostly young adults between the ages of 18 and 24, white, female, and overweight) who owned wearable fitness tracking devices completed a survey and took part in focus groups where they responded to questions regarding tracker features,

usage for physical activity, and motivation. Results showed that Fitbit was the most commonly used device, the most commonly used features were rewards/badges and notifications, and the most helpful ones were motivational cues and general health information. The authors claim that these preferences varied considerably by demographics, but the results were inconclusive (no statistical significance), which requires additional research in order to determine factors that led to increased engagement with difference device features. Another recent observational study [33] determined that wearable fitness tracking devices were able to accurately measure the level of physical activity of elderly people (70–90 years of age) in real-life settings.

[34] studied how college students are likely to use wearable fitness trackers and how they contribute towards increasing confidence and motivation for physical activity. Based on data collected from 67 participants who were enrolled at a Midwestern university, the authors found that females were 2.3 times more likely to use such trackers and that the availability of mobile apps associated with the trackers provided significant motivation for use. [35] reported a study based on 388 survey respondents, which found that users are generally satisfied with fitness trackers but believed that those devices were expensive. The top three health-related features that users preferred were heart-rate monitoring, a daily pedometer to measure the number of steps, and professional fitness tracking.

4.4 RESEARCH ON SECURITY OF MHEALTH TECHNOLOGY

Just as with any technology, privacy is of prime importance for all mobile healthcare technology. With advances in computational and storage capabilities, these devices capture massive amounts of sensitive health and fitness data automatically and persistently in real time from users so that ensuring their privacy and safety is of utmost importance. Moreover, the capabilities provided by most fitness trackers (and some mobile apps) for social networking and data sharing to their users also create additional risks and vulnerabilities for the data generated by these devices.

According to [36], the research literature in this area is sparse, but there are opportunities to learn from lessons in other communities, such as cybersecurity, as to how to reduce and prevent the potential risk of data breaches in mHealth technologies. According to the authors, issues of privacy and security remain an ongoing concern for researchers conducting mHealth studies, especially in sensitive medical areas such as obesity, cancer, and so on, where such technology is most often used for intervention purposes. [37] conducted an online survey among 212 fitness tracker users to understand their level of knowledge, attitudes, and behaviors related to the security and privacy associated with these devices. The findings showed that users knew much about the type of data collected by the trackers and were comfortable sharing their data with family and friends; however, they had little knowledge about how the tracked data are used and what steps to take to protect them from falling into the wrong hands. Thus, the authors concluded that much more awareness is required about issues regarding the privacy and safety of their own health and fitness data and also regarding how that data are stored and used by the manufacturer. A more recent study with 24 participants who evaluated the Fitbit Blaze device showed that most of the security and risk concerns arise from potentially fraudulent third-party applications and that users are justified in their concerns as these risks are very real [29]. [38] published findings from a survey of 361 Fitbit and Jawbone manufactured fitness trackers that showed how their demographics, privacy concerns, and technology skills impacted their data sharing behaviors and understanding of the sensitivity of their personal fitness information.

Several studies have explored vulnerabilities in different fitness trackers and their associated mobile applications. Probably the earliest security research on wearable fitness trackers focused on Fitbits [39], where the authors discovered several vulnerabilities via reverse engineering of some of their functionalities. Many later studies [40, 41] then discovered risks and vulnerabilities in the process by which data from the tracker is transmitted to the servers that can potentially reveal a user's sensitive information, like the encryption key stored in the tracker's memory in an unencrypted format (plain text). [42] compared the security features of data storage and transmission of nine different fitness trackers – namely, LG, Sony, Fitbit, Withings, Jawbone, Polar, Huawei, Garmin, and Acer. Their results showed that all devices use encrypted data, but the level of security for each is different. [43] analyzed potential security vulnerabilities of one of the most popular fitness tracking devices on the market in 2017 (name was not revealed) during the communication process when the data are shared with the manufacturer's servers and with third party applications.

4.5 CHALLENGES AND ISSUES IN FITNESS TRACKER RESEARCH

To date, fitness activity trackers and their benefits are not well understood, and that is in part due to data-related issues and conflicting research findings regarding their impacts on personal health. The primary challenge to conducting research on these devices is the availability of data, as many people stop using them after a short period of time. According to [44], about one-third of people who purchase fitness trackers stop using them within six months, and more than half eventually abandon them altogether. One reason behind this is loss of motivation [45]. People may buy these as technology 'fads' or because their friends or colleagues use them but then lose interest and motivation quickly because of time constraints posed by work and family commitments and in the absence of additional incentives. Another issue underlying motivation behind fitness tracker use is individual well-being. Well-being is not solely based on one's health condition; rather, it is driven by an ensemble of physical, social, emotional, and mental factors that create a sense of positivity about one's life. The perception of well-being differs from person to person, and typically a person undertakes tasks that will lead to a sense of accomplishment, personal fulfilment, mental or physical vitality, and social satisfaction [46]. So, although fitness trackers have the potential to improve one's health, people may experience negative outcomes such as technical issues or inaccuracies in measurements that can lead to dissatisfaction. Research has shown that self-quantifying mechanisms could reduce the enjoyment of partaking in health-related activities since they decrease their state of well-being [47].

Another associated issue or challenge with conducting research on fitness trackers is that not everyone who wears a fitness tracking device properly monitors their activity or uses it consistently. This leads to either significant losses of important tracking data or inaccuracies in the collected data. As a result, statistical analyses performed using these data can become invalid, thus rendering the interpretation of true impacts of these devices almost impossible. Fitness trackers possess the capabilities of collecting a tsunami of data, from physical activity levels, calories burnt, sleep patterns, and food and exercise, etc., so there is tremendous potential for obtaining rich insights not only about the impact of these devices but also regarding the different levels of relationships among different variables.

4.5.1 Potential Solutions

The obvious questions now are: (1) How will research on fitness trackers advance in the light of the above-mentioned challenges? (2) What can researchers do differently to ensure the success of their research on the topic? It is extremely important to find answers to these questions because, evidently, research can go a long way in helping people make informed decisions regarding the consistent usage of fitness tracking devices for their self-health management. Moreover, new research is required to advance and expand the health research community in this regard, thus providing new insights about the impact of these devices in different aspects on people's health and open the door for further opportunities.

So, we strive to provide potential solutions to the above two questions in the form of guidelines to help researchers pursue this area, based on our own experience in conducting research on fitness trackers. First and foremost, if subjects are involved in a study, particularly for longitudinal research designs that are meant to follow subjects over an extended period of time, the primary issue is to ensure that the subjects continue their participation throughout the duration of the study. For that, a key factor is motivation. Now, earlier studies have shown that standard incentives fail to provide the necessary motivation beyond a certain time period (about 3 – 6 months), so newer and more exciting incentives are called for that would be meaningful and fulfill a particular need. Previous research has shown that in cases where individuals receive corporate incentives (e.g., lower health insurance premiums), motivation is experienced at greater levels [48]. Often there are other underlying factors that can inspire motivation in an individual, such as behavioral factors like self-efficacy. People who are conscious about their own well-being and wish to lead healthy lifestyles on their own are more likely to have the necessary motivation to continue using these fitness trackers, even without any external incentives. In this regard, it might be advantageous for researchers to recruit such individuals for their research study via a widely circulated survey. But it is understandable that sometimes this is difficult to achieve, as the population from which participants are recruited may not have the required number of motivated participants, in which case, the researchers need to strive to create and offer satisfactory incentives to keep the participants sufficiently motivated to complete the study.

Some other ways to boost participant motivation is to provide them with very clear guidelines about the study and set expectations regarding how to fulfill all participation requirements. Not all individuals are equally tech-savvy, and hence detailed instructions about how to record their fitness data are essential. It is also a good practice to send periodic reminders to each participant, particularly in the beginning, to make sure that they have completed the necessary registration and sign-up steps. It is also critical to provide sufficient information to participants regarding how their data would be used for research – most importantly, how the data will be stored in password-protected computers and how the subjects' confidentiality and anonymity will be preserved while publishing the research. In this respect, the researchers can consider providing each participating subject with a copy of the IRB approval, as obtained from their institution, that outlines the research design protocol, associated risks and benefits, and privacy protection protocols. Health and fitness data are sensitive in nature, and people are rightly concerned about whether their data will be used appropriately and whether there are possibilities that they may be compromised in some way. One recent report [49] mentioned that health insurance companies can increase premiums based on fitness tracking data that they may have access to. Thus, transparency and clear guidelines at the beginning could potentially go a long way towards allaying general fears and concerns, thus leading to an increase in motivation for actively participating in the study.

The other challenging issue in the context of fitness tracker research is the quality of data obtained and the validity and accuracy of the results obtained by analyzing such data. Participants are often found to not sync their devices on a regular basis, thus creating 'holes' in the data that render longitudinal data analysis difficult. Coupled with this is the issue arising from missing data when individuals forget or refuse to record their activity data or leave the study early. In order to conduct statistical analysis, a reasonable sample size is essential (for instance, a minimum of 30 – 40). So, if that is not satisfied, the results and insights obtained will not be valid and useful. In fact, statistical inference theory says that the larger the sample size, more accurate and precise is the inference by providing a greater statistical power for the underlying hypothesis tests [50]. So, efforts are required on the part of the researchers to gather a reasonably large sample size, even beyond the minimum threshold of 30, for the inference to be statistically valid. In order to ensure this, it is thus extremely important to recruit participants appropriately (such that they are likely to continue) and keep them motivated and engaged enough in the study so that the data obtained are amenable to valid inference at the end.

Many research studies today use empirical and heuristic approaches for studying the impact of fitness trackers on people's health, such as weight loss, that are based on descriptive and summary statistics. These methods lack rigor, and the conclusions reached are usually restricted to the particular sample at hand and cannot be generalized to a larger population. This reduces the scope and significance of these research studies considerably, and all resources and efforts of the researchers are in vain. There are some studies in the literature, however, that are based on a systematically defined research design that have led to inference regarding associations and causal relationships that are interpretable in a meaningful way, but they also report the loss of participants in the middle of the study. [51] observed that out of 711 participants included in their research study, more than 25% had stopped using their Fitbit trackers after three months, and the average duration of tracker use was only 129 days (a little over six months). They concluded that technical, goal-related, and user experience factors were key determinants of sustained usage of fitness trackers. More and more studies of this kind are henceforth required to advance the research on this topic, which is gaining powerful ground day by day.

4.6 CONCLUSIONS AND FUTURE RESEARCH DIRECTIONS

The domain of mobile healthcare technology research has expanded significantly over the past six years since 2015–2016. It has been shown that of all the brands of wearable fitness tracking devices, the five most often used in research studies are Fitbit, Garmin, Misfit, Apple, and Polar [52]. Fitbit is used in twice as many validation studies as any other brands and is registered in clinical trial studies ten times more frequently than other brands. This is not surprising, given that Fitbit is the most popularly used wearable tracker today, with more than 100 million devices sold and 28 million users as of March 2020, and was the first one to start this ongoing movement of 'wearable fitness devices.'

Much of the current fitness tracker impact studies have considered either young adults (college-age population) or older adults. Further, most subjects involved in the studies were either overweight or suffered from some chronic conditions. Very few studies have covered a wider population with respect to age and a diverse group of individuals with different health conditions, from healthy ones to those with chronic and severe illnesses. Such studies are imperative to fully understand the impact of fitness trackers on the health and wellness of the general population.

Another issue is that the conclusions from many of the research studies are not definitive, and statistical significance of the results (differences between control and intervention groups, for instance) are not always clearly established. This raises some concerns regarding the benefits of mobile health technology, despite the fact that generally positive outcomes were noted for subjects using fitness trackers and mobile health apps in terms of improved health and fitness. Such outcomes are likely to create skepticism in the minds of people as to the value of these trackers and prevent more widespread adoption of these devices.

The privacy and security of mHealth devices is another potential area that is much less explored in research studies. Most of the existing scientific work focuses on identifying different types of vulnerabilities in fitness trackers, with relatively less progress reported in terms of the development of solutions to address these shortcomings. Because of its extreme importance, this presents researchers with rich opportunities to enhance the field by developing new security products for fitness trackers and mobile apps and increase the security of the devices so that consumers can use them with more confidence.

Lastly, it should be noted that the overview of research presented in this chapter is not necessarily exhaustive. In particular, an abundance of scientific studies was published since 2019, and new studies are coming out on a daily basis, given that this is a fast-developing field. But we strived to ensure that a broad spectrum of research on mobile healthcare technology is covered here that will provide researchers with a deeper understanding of the current breadth of work done in this area and will help lay the groundwork for future studies, as outlined above.

NOTES

1 https://fitbug.com/
2 www.withings.com/us/en/watches

REFERENCES

1. '*Pedometers help people stay active; Stanford study finds.*' Website: http://med.stanford.edu/news/all-news/2007/11/pedometers-help-people-stay-active-stanford-study-finds.html. Retrieved on February 2, 2019.
2. Gierisch, J.G., Goode, A.P., Allen, K.D., Batch, B.C., Shaw, R.J. (2015). The Impact of Pedometers on Chronic Conditions – A Review of Reviews, *White paper, Department of Veterans Affairs*, Durham, NC.

3. Shimon, J., Petlichkoff, L.M. (2009). Impact of Pedometer use and self-regulation strategies on junior high school physical education students' daily step counts. *Journal of Physical Activity and Health*, 6(2): 178–184.
4. Cayir, Y., Aslan, S.M., Akturk, Z. (2015). The effect of pedometer use on physical activity and body weight in obese women. *European Journal of Sport Science*, 15(4): 351–356.
5. Stiglbauer, B., Weber, S., Batinic, B. (2019). Does your health really benefit from using a self-tracking device? Evidence from a longitudinal randomized control trial. *Computers in Human Behavior*, 94, 131–139.
6. Schaben, J.A., Furness, S. (2018). Investing in college students: the role of fitness tracker. *Digital Health*, 2018 Apr 4, 4: 2055207618766800. DOI: 10.1177/2055207618766800
7. Brickwood, K., Watson, G., O'Brien, J., Williams, A.D. (2019). Consumer-Based Wearable Activity Trackers Increase Physical Activity Participation: Systematic Review and Meta-Analysis. *Journal of Medical Internet Research (JMIR) Mhealth Uhealth*, 7(4):e11819.
8. Silveira, S.L., Baird, J.F., Motl, R.W. (2021). Rates, patterns, and correlates of fitness tracker use among older adults with multiple sclerosis. Disability and Health Journal, 14(1), DOI: https://doi.org/10.1016/j.dhjo.2020.100966.
9. Solon, O. (2015). Wearable Technology Creeps into The Workplace. *Bloomberg.com*. Link: www.bloomberg.com/news/articles/2015-08- 07/wearable-technology-creeps-into-the-workplace. Retrieved on July 23, 2021.
10. Olson, P. (2016). Fitbit's Game Plan for Making Your Company Healthy. *Forbes*. Link: www.forbes.com/sites/parmyolson/2016/01/08/fitbit-wearables-corporate-wellness/. Retrieved on July 23, 2021.
11. Clubbs, B.H., Gray, N., Madlock, P. (2021). Using the theory of planned behavior and the technology acceptance model to analyze a university employee fitness tracker program with financial incentive, *Journal of Communication in Healthcare*, 14:2, 149–162, DOI: 10.1080/17538068.2020.1864614
12. Giddens, L., Leidner, D., Gonzalez, E. (2017). The role of Fitbits in corporate wellness programs: Does step count matter? In *Proceedings of the 50*th *Hawaii International Conference on System Sciences (HICSS)*, January 4–7, 2017, Waikoloa, Hawaii.
13. Friess, M., Stukenberg, E. (2016). A quantitative pilot study on the use of a fitness tracker in the preventative management of employees at risk of chronic disease in a health care facility. *Online Journal of Nursing Informatics*, 19(3):1.
14. Finkelstein, E.A., Haaland, B.A., Bilger, M., et al. (2016). Effectiveness of activity trackers with and without incentives to increase physical activity (TRIPPA): a randomized controlled trial. *The Lancet: Diabetes & Endocrinology*, 4(12): 983–995.

15. Jakicic, J.M., Davis, K.K., Rogers, R.J., et al (2016). Effect of Wearable Technology Combined with a Lifestyle Intervention on Long-term Weight Loss: The IDEA Randomized Clinical Trial. *Journal of the American Medical Association (JAMA)*, 316(11): 1161–1171.
16. Kernebeck, S., Busse, T. S., Böttcher, M. D., Weitz, J., Ehlers, J., & Bork, U. (2020). Impact of mobile health and medical applications on clinical practice in gastroenterology. *World Journal of Gastroenterology*, 26(29), 4182–4197. https://doi.org/10.3748/wjg.v26.i29.4182.
17. Beratarrechea, A., Lee, A.G., Willner, J.M., Eiman Jahangir, Ciapponi, A., Rubinstein, A. (2014). *Telemedicine and e-Health*, 20(1): 75–82. http://doi.org/10.1089/tmj.2012.0328
18. Stork, M.J., Bell, E.G., Jung, M.E. (2021). Examining the Impact of a Mobile Health App on Functional Movement and Physical Fitness: Pilot Pragmatic Randomized Controlled Trial. *Journal of Medical Internet Research (JMIR) Mhealth Uhealth*, 9(5):e24076, doi: 10.2196/24076
19. Ghose, A. (2021). Do Health Apps really make us healthier? *Harvard Business Review*, May 7, 2021. Link: https://hbr.org/2021/05/do-health-apps-really-make-us-healthier. Retrieved on September 6, 2021.
20. Yerrakalva, D., Yerrakalva, D., Hajna S., Griffin, S. (2019). Effects of Mobile Health App Interventions on Sedentary Time, Physical Activity, and Fitness in Older Adults: Systematic Review and Meta-Analysis. *Journal of Medical Internet Research*, 21(11):e14343. DOI: 10.2196/14343
21. Iribarren, S.J., Akande, T.O., Kamp, K.J., Barry, D., Kader, Y.G., Suelzer, E. (2021). Effectiveness of Mobile Apps to Promote Health and Manage Disease: Systematic Review and Meta-analysis of Randomized Controlled Trials. *Journal of Medical Internet Research (JMIR) Mhealth Uhealth*, 9(1):e21563. doi: 10.2196/21563
22. Byambasuren, O., Sanders, S., Beller, E. et al. (2018). Prescribable mHealth apps identified from an overview of systematic reviews. *npj Digital Medicine* 1(12).
23. Ting, D.S.W., Carin, L., Dzau, V., Wong, T.Y (2020). Digital technology and COVID-19. *Nature Medicine*, 26: 459–461.
24. Singh, H.J.L., Couch, D., Yap, K. (2020). Mobile Health Apps That Help With COVID-19 Management: Scoping Review. *Journal of Medical Internet Research Nursing*, 3(1), e20596. https://doi.org/10.2196/20596.
25. Almalki M., Giannicchi A. (2021). Health Apps for Combating COVID-19: Descriptive Review and Taxonomy *Journal of Medical Internet Research (JMIR) Mhealth Uhealth*, 9(3): e24322, doi: 10.2196/24322
26. Laranjo L., Ding D., Heleno, B., et al (2021). Do smartphone applications and activity trackers increase physical activity in adults? Systematic review,

meta-analysis and meta-regression. *British Journal of Sports Medicine*, 55(8):422–432.

27. Hills, A. P., Mokhtar, N., Byrne, N. M. (2014). Assessment of physical activity and energy expenditure: an overview of objective measures. *Frontiers in nutrition*, 1, 5. https://doi.org/10.3389/fnut.2014.00005.
28. Park, W., Lee, V.J., Ku, B., Tanaka, H. (2014). Effect of walking speed and placement position interactions in determining the accuracy of various newer pedometers, *Journal of Exercise Science & Fitness*, 2(1): 31–37.
29. Orlosky, J., Ezenwoye, O., Yates, H., Besenyi, G. (2019). A look at the security and privacy of Fitbit as a health activity tracker. In *Proceedings of 2019 ACM Southeast Conference*, pages: 241–244, April 2019, Kennesaw (GA).
30. Feehan, L. M., Geldman, J., Sayre, E. C., Park, C., Ezzat, A. M., Yoo, J. Y., Hamilton, C. B., Li, L. C. (2018). Accuracy of Fitbit Devices: Systematic Review and Narrative Syntheses of Quantitative Data, *Journal of Medical Internet Research* (JMIR); mHealth and uHealth, 6(8), e10527. Doi: https://doi.org/10.2196/10527
31. Kroll, R.R., Boyd, J.G., Maslove, D.M. (2016). Accuracy of a Wrist-Worn Wearable Device for Monitoring Heart Rates in Hospital Inpatients: A Prospective Observational Study, *Journal of Medical Internet Research* (JMIR);18(9): e253. doi: 10.2196/jmir.6025
32. Lewis, Z.H., Pritting, L., Picazo, A.L., Tucker, M.J-M. (2020). The utility of wearable fitness trackers and implications for increased engagement: An exploratory, mixed methods observational study. Digital Health, 2020 Jan-Dec 6: 2055207619900059. DOI: 10.1177/2055207619900059
33. Martinato, M., Lorenzoni, G., Zanchi, T., Bergamin, A., Buratin, A., Azzolina, D., Gregori, D. (2021). Usability and Accuracy of a Smartwatch for the Assessment of Physical Activity in the Elderly Population: Observational Study, *Journal of Medical Internet Research* (JMIR) Mhealth Uhealth; 9(5): e20966. doi: 10.2196/20966
34. Kinney, D. (2017). College Students Use and Perceptions of Wearable Fitness Trackers and Mobile Health Apps, *Doctoral dissertation, University of Cincinnati*. OhioLINK Electronic Theses and Dissertations Center. Link: http://rave.ohiolink.edu/etdc/view?acc_num=ucin1504798862580571
35. Jia, Y., Wang, W., Wen, D., Liang, L., Gao, L., Lei, J. (2018). Perceived user preferences and usability evaluation of mainstream wearable devices for health monitoring, PeeJ, 6(7): e5350. Doi: 10.7717/peerj.5350
36. Arora, S., Yttri, J., & Nilse, W. (2014). Privacy and Security in Mobile Health (mHealth) Research. *Alcohol research: current reviews*, 36(1), 143–151.
37. Gabriele, S., Chiasson, S. (2020). Understanding fitness tracker users' security and privacy knowledge, attitudes and behaviors. In *Proceedings of the 2020*

CHI Conference on Human Factors in Computing Systems, Honolulu (HI), April 2020, pages: 1–12.

38. Vitak J., Liao Y., Kumar P., Zimmer M., Kritikos K. (2018). Privacy Attitudes and Data Valuation Among Fitness Tracker Users. In: *Chowdhury G., McLeod J., Gillet V., Willett P. (eds) Transforming Digital Worlds. iConference 2018. Lecture Notes in Computer Science*, Vol. 10766, pages: 229–239. Springer, Cham.
39. Rahman, M., Carbunar, B., Banik, M. (2013). Fit and Vulnerable: Attacks and Defenses for a Health Monitoring Device. In *Proceedings of IEEE Symposium on Security and Privacy (IEEE S&P)*, Vol. 34, May 2013, San Francisco (CA).
40. Cyr, B., Horn, W., Miao, D., Specter, M. (2013). Security Analysis of Wearable Fitness Trackers (Fitbit); Technical Report, *Massachusetts Institute of Technology (MIT)*: Cambridge, MA, USA.
41. Schellevis, M., Jacobs, B., Meijer, C., de Ruiter, J. (2016). Getting Access to your Own Fitbit Data; *Radboud University: Nijmegen*, The Netherlands.
42. Clausing, E., Schiefer, M., Lösche, U. (2015). Internet of Things Security Evaluation of nine Fitness Trackers; *Technical Report; AV TEST: The Independent IT-Security Institute:* Magdeburg, Germany.
43. Mendoza, F., Alonso, L., López, A., & and Patricia Arias Cabarcos, D. (2018). Assessment of Fitness Tracker Security: A Case of Study. *Proceedings (MDPI)*, 2(19), 1235. doi:10.3390/proceedings2191235
44. Pai, A. (2014). Survey: One third of wearable device owners stopped using them within six months. *Mobile Health News*, Link: www.mobihealthnews.com/31697/survey-one-third-of-wearable-device-owners-stopped-using-them-within-six-months, published on April 3, 2014. Retrieved on November 10, 2021.
45. Rupp, M.A., Michaelis, J.R., McConnell, D.S., and Smither, J.A. (2018). The Role of Individual Differences on Perceptions of Wearable Fitness Device Trust, Usability, and Motivational Impact. *Applied Ergonomics*, 70: 77-87.
46. Naci, H. and Ioannidis, J.P.A. (2015). Evaluation of Wellness Determinants and Interventions by Citizen Scientists. *Journal of American Medical Association*, 314(2): 121–122.
47. Etkin, J. (2016). The Hidden Cost of Personal Quantification. *Journal of Consumer Research*, 42(6): 967–984.
48. Gonzalez, E., Mitra, S. (2019). Wearable technologies: The motivational impacts on individual well-being, In *Proceedings of 25th America's Conference on Information Systems (AMCIS)*, Cancun, Mexico, August 15-19, 2019.
49. ABC News (2019). What if your fitness tracker was used to set your health insurance premiums? The Conversation. Link: www.abc.net.au/news/2019-07-08/fitness-tracker-used-to-set-health-insurance-premiums/11287126, published on July 7, 2019. Retrieved on November 20, 2021.

50. Cox, D. (2006). Principles of Statistical Inference, Cambridge University Press, 1st edition.
51. Hermsen, S., Moons, J., Kerkhof, P., Wiekens, C., De Groot, M. (2017). Determinants for Sustained Use of an Activity Tracker: Observational Study. *Journal of Medical Internet Research* (JMIR); mHealth and uHealth, 5(10), e164. https://doi.org/10.2196/mhealth.7311.
52. Henriksen, A., Haugen Mikalsen, M., Woldaregay, A. Z., Muzny, M., Hartvigsen, G., Hopstock, L. A., & Grimsgaard, S. (2018). Using Fitness Trackers and Smartwatches to Measure Physical Activity in Research: Analysis of Consumer Wrist-Worn Wearables. *Journal of Medical Internet Research*, 20(3), e110. https://doi.org/10.2196/jmir.9157.

CHAPTER 5

mHealth Technology and Social Media

5.1 INTRODUCTION

Social media, loosely defined as interactive computer-based technologies meant to connect people via the creation and sharing of information and ideas [1], is a huge part of the society today. Social media typically contains user-generated content, such as text posts and comments, photos, and videos stored in a user's profile, that is designed and maintained by a social media organization. Users then interact and communicate with each other and form groups with individuals they know, thus creating communities through social networking. Social media thus differs from traditional media like newspapers (paper-based) and television (electronic) in many ways, including quality, reach, frequency, interactivity, usability, and performance [2]. Some of the most popular social media websites with over 100 million registered users today are Facebook, YouTube, Instagram, Twitter, Tumblr, LinkedIn, Snapchat, Pinterest, and Reddit, to name a few. Almost all these websites can be accessed by an individual from any web-based technology, such as a computer desktop or laptop, as well as a mobile device, such as a smartphone or tablet. Specific mobile applications or apps are also available on smartphones today to access such sites easily with the tap of a button, resulting in widespread access and use.

In this chapter, we provide a brief overview of social media and its impact on mobile healthcare technology. The rest of the chapter is organized as follows. Section 5.2 outlines currently available social media platforms and

DOI: 10.1201/9780429428449-5

applications, and Section 5.3 describes the role of social media in mHealth, along with the most popular social fitness apps and their potential advantages and disadvantages. Section 5.4 provides a summary of currently existing research on the impact of social media and social networking on different aspects of mobile healthcare, and finally our overall conclusions are presented in Section 5.5.

5.2 DIFFERENT TYPES OF SOCIAL MEDIA

Figure 5.1 shows a snapshot of these common social media sites and the corresponding apps available on a mobile device.

Social media use is widespread today. Individuals typically use social media to express themselves, discuss their interests, connect with friends and family members, and grow their careers. Companies are also increasingly leveraging the wide outreach of these platforms for marketing purposes, such as increasing brand awareness, generating traffic, building loyalty of current customers, and creating new customers. In fact, according to a recent blog post, over 88% of business are now using social media for marketing [3]. The list of social media platforms continues to grow, and existing platforms keep adding new features and tools to increase their functionalities and attract more users.

Broadly speaking, there are nine different types of social media [4], which we describe below along with brief details about the most popular and well-known platforms for each type:

1) *Social networks* – probably the first and most popular type of social media today, such sites are used mainly to connect with people and share stories and interests. Business can also use these sites for social

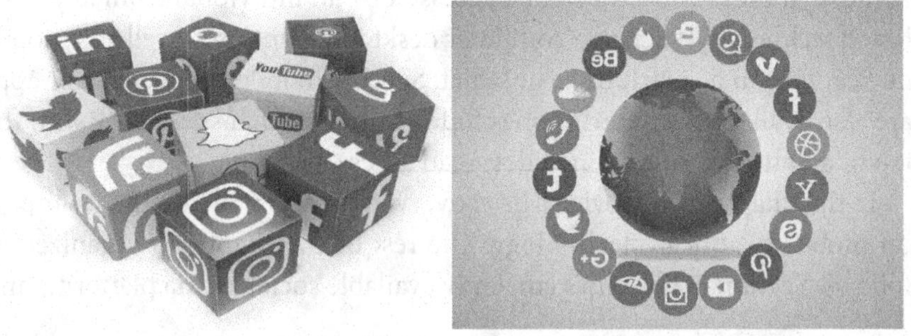

FIGURE 5.1 Popular social media platforms available today. (License: CC.)

awareness of their brands, relationship building, customer service, and lead generation and conversion. Example of well-known social networking sites include Facebook (2.82 billion active users as of March 31, 2021), Twitter (199 million daily users as of 2021), and LinkedIn (160 million users in U.S. alone as of 2021), of which the latter mainly emphasizes career-related networking. On all these networks, users can communicate with each other through simple actions such as chatting, posting content (text, pictures, videos), re-sharing content posted by others, reacting to and commenting on others' posts, private messaging, tagging, and hashtagging.[1] Moreover, Facebook and Twitter now allow live streams of events that can be watched worldwide. All of these functionalities thus provide considerable flexibility in how users can use such platforms that have also significantly contributed to the growth of the user population. Figure 5.2 shows a typical Facebook 'chat' and Twitter page interface.

2) *Media sharing networks* – these sites allow users to find and share photos, videos, live videos, and other types of media. The most popular platforms providing these services include Instagram (1 billion monthly active users worldwide as of 2021), Snapchat (293 million daily active users worldwide as of 2021), Flickr (112 million registered members as of 2015), and YouTube (2.3 billion users worldwide as of 2021). Instagram provides a visual feed where users can post photos and videos with captions. They can also post live video or create Instagram stories[2] that stay active on the user's page for 24 hours. Unlike social networking sites, Instagram does not allow direct

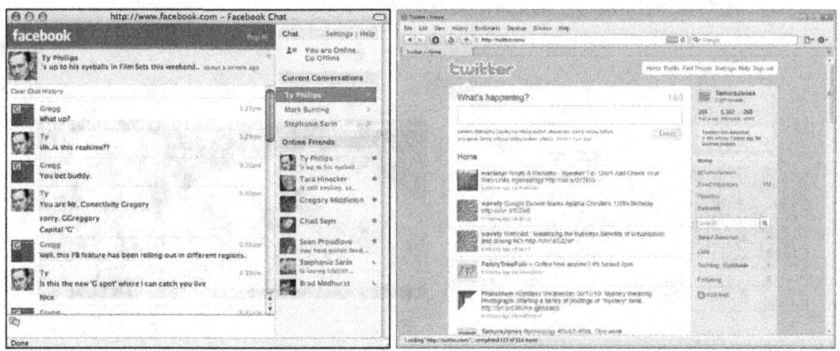

FIGURE 5.2 Facebook 'chat' and Twitter interface. (License: CC.)

sharing of links in posts (which must be posted under a user's bio), but it allows users to communicate and interact with each other via comments, tags, likes, or direct messaging. Launched in September 2011, Snapchat is a multimedia messaging service wherein users could share short chats or photos for a short time before they became unavailable; however now these are mostly available for 24 hours to the recipients. YouTube is today probably the most popular social media platform offering video sharing service; it started in February 2005 and is currently owned by Google. It is the second most visited website today, with more than 1 billion hours of video watching on a daily basis [5]. Since its birth, YouTube has considerably expanded its platform to offer mobile apps and allow streaming of movies, music videos, short films, educational videos, audio recordings, video blogs (vlogs), and much more. Figure 5.3 shows a typical Instagram (chat) and You Tube and page interface. Flickr, founded in 2004, is a photo and video sharing service that also provides an online community for sharing with others. Although primarily meant for amateur and professional photographers to showcase their work, Flickr eventually reached the general public, although its popularity has declined significantly with the advent of Instagram and Pinterest.

3) *Bookmarking and Content Curation networks* – Pinterest (478 million active monthly users globally as of 2021) and Flipboard are social media platforms that help users find, share, and discuss a variety of latest trends in different areas such as fashion, food, travel, news, entertainment, and so on. Pinterest, launched in December 2009, allows image sharing and the discovery and saving of information found online using images, animated GIFs, and videos (via 'visual' searches). Pinterest consists of a board that consists of different

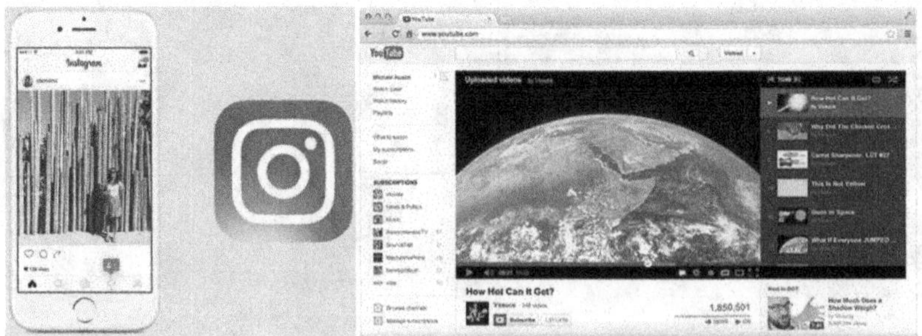

FIGURE 5.3 Instagram mobile and YouTube interface. (License: CC.)

images (referred to as 'pins') uploaded by a user or linked from a website and shared with others. Similarly, Flipboard offers users a platform to aggregate content from social media, news feeds, image sharing websites, and other outlets in a 'magazine' format that can be saved and shared with others. Relatively less used that other social media sites, Flipboard had reported that there were 28 million magazines created by users in March 2016 (no recent data found). Figure 5.4 shows a typical Pinterest page interface.

4) *Discussion Forums* – social media platforms like Reddit, Quora, and Digg fall in this category, where users are mainly interested in finding, sharing, and discussing different kinds of information, news, and opinions. Answers to common questions can be found also in various domains and hence are informative and useful. These platforms are also very useful for business marketing campaigns (like advertising), as they have a massive number of users and widespread reach.
5) *Consumer review networks* – social media sites like Yelp, Zomato, and TripAdvisor lets users leave reviews and comments about different services, products, and brands that they have used. These include restaurants, hotels, bars, beauty salons, dentists, plumbing services,

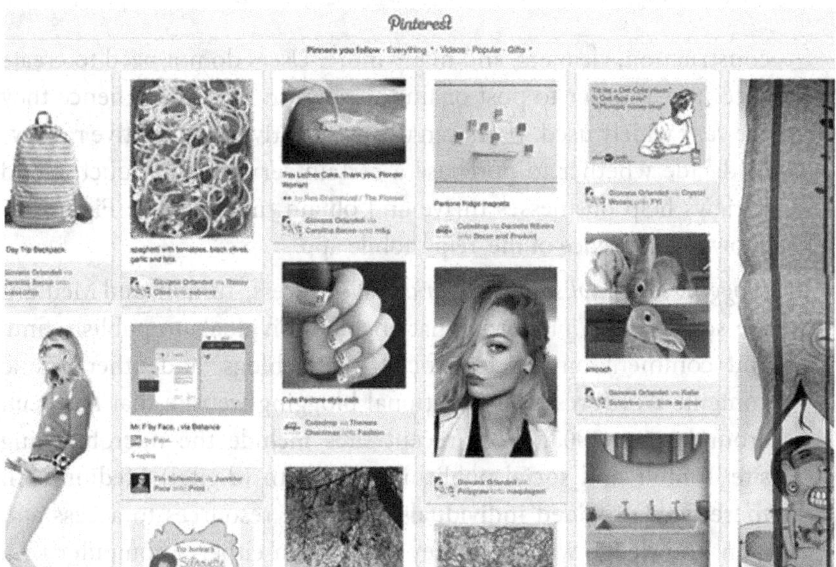

FIGURE 5.4 Pinterest interface. (License: CC.)

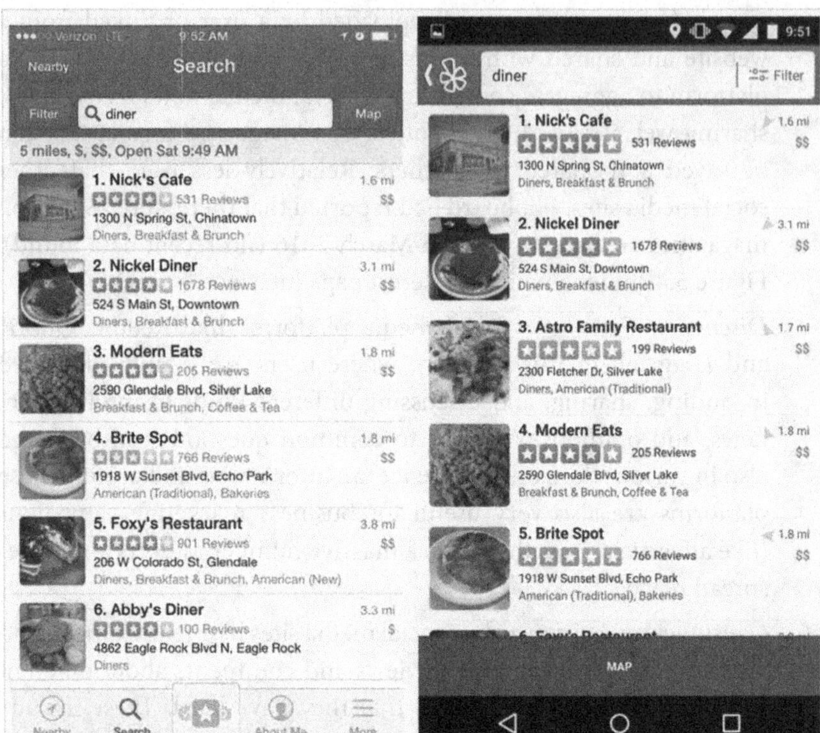

FIGURE 5.5 Yelp (mobile) interface. (License: CC.)

construction, cleaners, and many more. Users do not need to create accounts in order to post or find reviews in these sites; hence they are very widely used. Users can use the positive and negative reviews to decide whether to purchase a certain service or product. Good reviews help businesses thrive and obtain more clients. Figure 5.5 shows an interface of the Yelp mobile app.

6) *Blogging and publishing networks* – WordPress, Tumblr, and Medium are social media platforms that enable individuals to publish, find, and comment on articles, social media blogs, and other online content. WordPress is a traditional blogging website that has been around since 2003. More recent sites include the microblogging site Tumblr and social publishing platform (digital) Medium. All these have provided individuals with rich resources to access and gain knowledge whenever they wish, from either a computer or a mobile device, and foster research, discovery, and growth that were

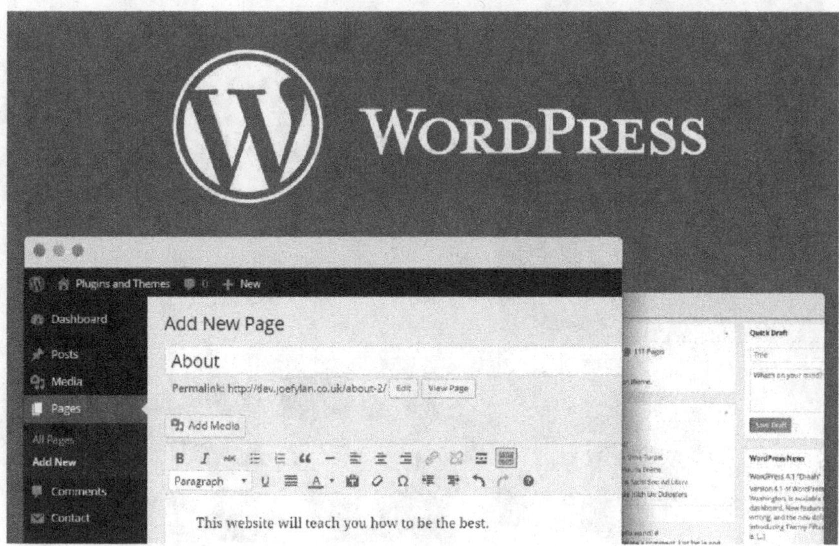

FIGURE 5.6 WordPress interface. (License: CC.)

not possible before these platforms were launched. Figure 5.6 shows an interface of the WordPress platform.

7) *Social shopping networks* – the growth of online technologies is in part largely driven by online shopping (also referred to as e-commerce). Social shopping networks provide information about the latest trends in the market in different areas, shopping tips, and reviews of items that are helpful to customers before making purchases. Moreover, these sites enable people to follow different brands and share interesting facts about them. Some common platforms in this category include Etsy, Polyvore, and Fancy. Etsy, in particular, specializes in selling handmade and ethnic items and craft supplies such as jewelry, bags, art, toys, clothes, furniture, etc. Even online retailers like Amazon let customers provide reviews and ratings of items they have purchased, which can be read and taken into account by other new customers while buying similar products. These sites have taken online shopping to a whole different level by taking them more engaging via social elements. Figure 5.7 shows an interface of the Etsy platform.
8) *Interest-based networks* – there are some specialized social media sites that provide individuals the opportunity to connect and interact with others who share similar interests and/or hobbies. Some

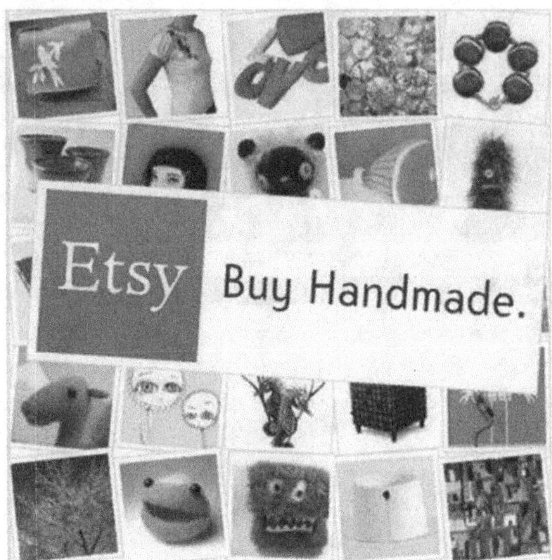

FIGURE 5.7 Etsy interface. (License: CC.)

examples of platforms belonging to this category include Goodreads (for books), Houzz (architecture home design and decorating), and Last.fm (music). These networks also help businesses to engage with their audience and create brand awareness online.

9) *Instant messaging (IM) networks* – WhatsApp is probably the most popular instant messaging service today used mostly on smartphones and other mobile devices equipped with internet connections. This application can be used to send texts, photos, documents, and audio and video recordings to other users, make phone and video calls, and create groups and communities. Launched in January 2010, WhatsApp was purchased by Facebook in 2014 and has over 2 billion users worldwide as of February 2020. WhatsApp has very quickly become the primary means of internet communication in multiple locations, including Latin America, the Indian subcontinent, and large parts of Europe and Africa [6]. Although messaging services are integrated with most social media platforms today, some of the most popular instant messaging services apart from WhatsApp are Facebook messenger, WeChat,[3] QQ Messenger,[4] Telegram,[5] and Snapchat. Figure 5.8 shows an interface of the WhatsApp platform on a smartphone.

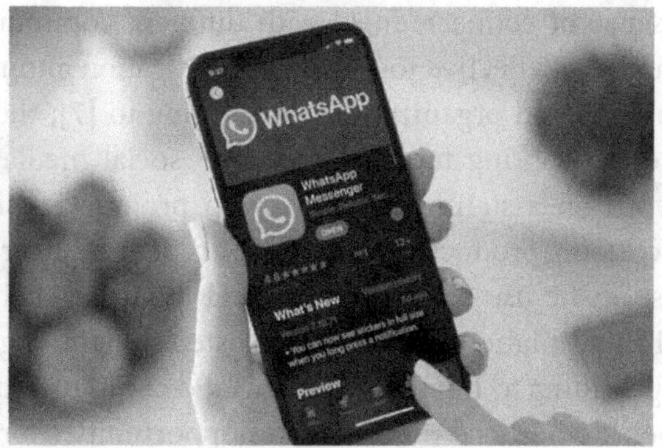

FIGURE 5.8 WhatsApp interface. (License: CC.)

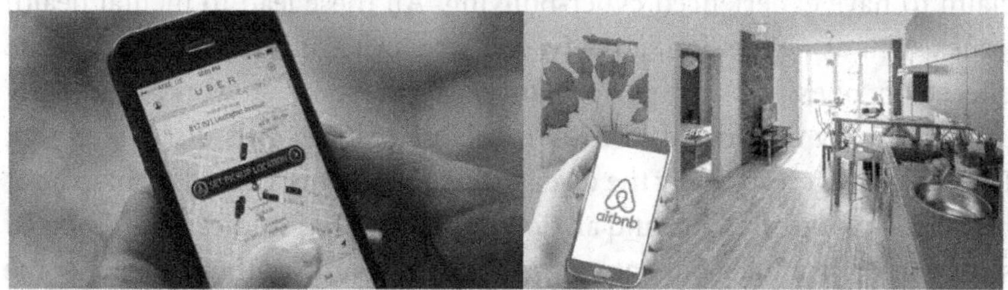

FIGURE 5.9 Uber and Airbnb (mobile) interfaces. (License: CC.)

10) *Other miscellaneous networks* – there are also other types of social media sites that do not clearly belong to any of the above eight categories. 'Sharing economy networks' provide people with a platform to advertise, find, buy, sell, and trade products and services. Some popular sites that facilitate these activities are Airbnb (accommodations), Uber (rideshare and food delivery), and TaskRabbit (labor). Finally, there are 'anonymous' networks like Whisper, Ask.fm, etc. that are meant for people to vent, gossip, and follow others in an anonymous manner. Most articles advise people against using these websites, as there are often legal issues and consequences associated with these. Figure 5.9 shows the mobile interfaces of the Uber and Airbnb platforms.

5.2.1 Impact of Social Media on Society

Researchers have reported both positive and negative impacts of social media use. Social media provides people with an easily accessible pathway to develop a sense of connectedness with different communities, real or online, and can be an effective tool for communication and marketing for different businesses and organizations. According to [7], the various collaboration and networking tools provided by social media have helped students to work on assignments and group projects outside of school hours, thus increasing productivity as well as academic performance. Some instructors also make use of blogs and social media in their classrooms, both in K – 12 and higher education, to foster student engagement and active learning, leading to improved writing and communication skills.

On the other hand, social media creates opportunities for online fraud (stealing of one's identity and data), online harassment and cyber-bullying. According to a recent survey in the U.S., 69% of seventh grade students claim to have experienced cyber-bullying. All these lead to mental health issues such as depression, anxiety, and stress that in turn lead to adverse effects on one's life and performance in school or at work. One early research study conducted in 2009 involving teenage girls discovered that Facebook usage, especially the discussion of problems, caused them to be at higher risk for depression and anxiety [8]. Moreover, studies have reported strong addictive behaviors among adolescents and youth regarding some types of social media usage, like gaming, which have been known to cause disruptions in sleep patterns, weight and exercise levels, and more prominently in their academic performance. According to some recent research studies, long hours spent on mobile devices have shown a positive relationship with weight gain and a decrease in physical activity levels in teenagers, while a strong negative relationship with GPA [9, 10]. Moreover, such behaviors are also known to take away family and personal time, often leading to the development of anti-social behavior [11].

Just as with young children and adolescents, negative impacts of social media are also prevalent among the adult population. A study by Dr. Becker at Michigan State University [12] found that people who engage more with social media via gaming and texting were significantly more likely to suffer from depression, anxiety, and stress. A recent survey [13] showed that out of 7,000 mothers, 42% of those who used the photo-sharing social media site Pinterest reported suffering from stress. Apart from these emotional problems, social media is also increasingly being used to carry out criminal activities. These range from financial scams to drug dealing, human trafficking, and terrorism. According to a report by Weimann [14], cyberspace, and social media in particular, has been used extensively by terrorists to communicate and plan attacks, spread their propaganda, and raise funds as well as to recruit new members even from before 9/11. Cybercrimes, such as false messaging via social media and scams to steal money, are also skyrocketing, and they are creating extensive damage owing to the massive reach of social media platforms (mostly with over several million users).

It is thus probably advisable for everybody to use social media in a controlled and balanced manner so as to reap its benefits without affecting their own physical and mental health, and in particular, the usage by young people must be supervised and monitored by their parents.

5.3 THE ROLE OF SOCIAL MEDIA IN MHEALTH

Given the huge user base on social media today, it is easy to understand that it is able to provide an effective and accessible platform for mobile healthcare today. Healthcare organizations are increasingly leveraging the power of social networking sites to reach their patients and connect them with healthcare providers and online communities of other patients for different purposes, from helping them manage their own health to seek help and advice from both medical professionals and from other patients with similar health conditions and diagnoses. WebMD is a popular health information services website that publishes content regarding different aspects of healthcare as well as helps patients connect with doctors and other medical personnel. Towards the end of 2016, WebMD recorded an average of 179.5 million unique users per month, and 3.63 billion page visits per quarter [15].

According to a Health Research Institute survey [16], 42% consumers are using social media today to access consumer reviews of treatments, physicians, and hospitals, and 20% have joined a health-related forum or community. However, the most interesting finding from the survey was that more than 80% of consumers in the age group 18–24 years use social media to use and share health information, and 40% mentioned that their healthcare decisions were influenced by social media. Moreover, more than 700 of the 5,000 U.S. hospitals have a social media presence to enhance their marketing efforts and establish effective communication with stakeholders.

Many corporate wellness programs are also encouraging their employees to use fitness trackers (often with incentive such as lower cost of the devices) in order to participate in individual and group tasks and challenges related to different types of physical activities for the purpose of maintaining a healthy lifestyle as well as lowering insurance costs for both the employer and the employees. Recent studies showed that two companies, Dayton Regional Transit Authority and Springbuk, deployed Fitbit as part of their organizational wellness program and witnessed healthcare cost savings and improved health outcomes for their employees [17].

5.3.1 Most Popular Social Health and Fitness Apps

Most fitness trackers like Fitbit, provide the opportunity to connect with friends, family members, neighbors, and co-workers and share physical activity statistics with each other. Often, this is considered a way to obtain support in order to be successful in maintaining or achieving a healthy lifestyle. Competing with and receiving accolades for meeting activity goals can go a long way towards providing the motivation to an individual that is needed to keep him or her continuing to achieve health goals. Figure 5.10 below shows a typical mobile app dashboard of the popular fitness device Fitbit where the 'Friends' tab represents the social networking aspect. Apple Watch also supports social media apps like Twitter and Instagram by syncing with an iPhone, as shown in Figure 5.11. However, Apple Watch does not offer specialized networking capabilities with other Apple Watch users like Fitbit.

Some other common social fitness apps in use today are briefly discussed below [18]:

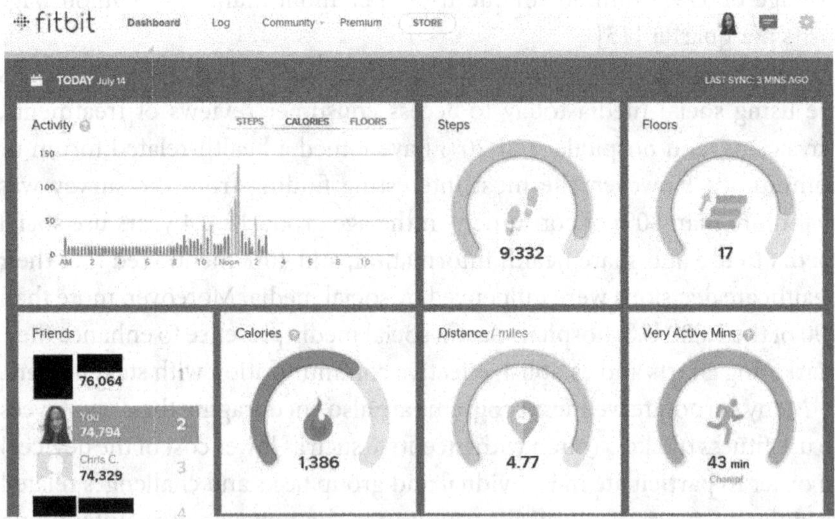

FIGURE 5.10 A typical dashboard interface of a fitness tracker that shows the 'social networking' aspect (Fitbit). (License: CC.)

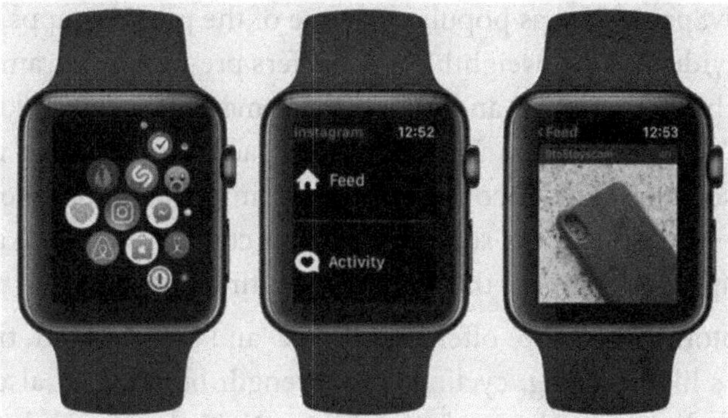

FIGURE 5.11 Instagram and Twitter apps and feeds on an Apple Watch. (License: CC.)

a) Pantheon: This app is built for helping teams to get fit together. Rather than giving the same goal to everyone, it gives an award to whoever gets the most steps, and it also recognizes each person based on their level of effort and creates goals based on their activity, exercise, meditation, and ability to work together with team members.

b) Nike Run Club: This app is a run tracker produced by Nike to help a person run better. Nike has running coaches and guided runs to help each person pace himself/herself or learn new ways of running. The competition is in the form of a leaderboard where everyone can keep track of the number of miles run by the others in real time. When a person goes for a run, all of their contacts in the network are notified.

c) Strava: This app is designed for mainly runners and cyclists and tracks how an individual runs or bikes. This app also lets people post routes, which are known as Segments in the Strava community. Whoever can complete a segment the fastest becomes 'king' of that segment. This leads to intense competition among runners and cyclists in different places as people work hard to overtake each other.

d) MyFitnessPal:[6] This is one of the most popular mobile health apps today to monitor one's diet. One can scan the barcodes of food items in the app so that it can track calorie intake, macronutrient breakdown, water intake, and weight goals. It is can also monitor exercises and track the number of calories burnt.

e) BodySpace:[7] Not as popular as some of the previous apps, this helps individuals track weightlifting. It offers pre-built programs, or users can build their own and obtain a summary of their workouts at the end of each session. Fitness coaches are also available to provide personalized guidance and effective training methods. The app offers a community aspect so that users can connect with one another to compete or compare their exercise routines.

f) Peloton:[8] This app offers both live and on-demand training in areas like running, cycling, and strength building. It also provides guided yoga, cardio, and stretching activities and even has workout equipment, accessories, and apparel for users to purchase. A recent addition to the app is a new feature called 'Tags' where the user can do group workouts. Joining a Tags group will let the user see what kinds of workouts their friends are engaging in and hence can encourage each other to stay fit and provide recommendations.

g) Shred:[9] This app provides the user with the opportunity to work out at home or at the gym with different types of training programs and video classes. There is also a community feature of this app that promotes networking with friends and influencers for additional inspiration and motivation. Friends can also engage in workout competitions if desired to provide extra encouragement to those who need it to remain active and healthy.

5.3.2 Advantages and Disadvantages

Social media has its benefits like wide outreach, access, and connectivity, and the mobile health apps that leverage these have become popular very quickly as a result. Friends and family provide motivation to each other to attain health goals and lead healthier lives. On the other hand, by following influencers, athletes, and other leaders of the leaders' boards, users get a chance to improve on their routines and post questions or queries. Moreover, information and resources available through these apps have proved very helpful, whether they are obtained from blogs, friends, trainers, or expert coaches with no need to visit a gym. The recent COVID-19 driven lockdown had closed down gyms and training facilities all around the world, which had adversely impacted people's health and fitness regimes. Fitness trackers and mobile health, especially with the added advantage of networking with others, proved invaluable in those times to many people in maintaining a healthy lifestyle amid numerous restrictions and constraints.

As with all technology, there are certain disadvantages associated with using social fitness apps. The primary shortcoming is that many measurements captured by these apps (like daily steps, calorie intake, etc.) are not always 100% accurate. Often, different apps or trackers provide different values, which can be very confusing to users. This can demotivate some users to stop using them altogether. Sometimes people post misinformation about diets and fitness, which can affect others' health if that information is not particularly checked and verified [19]. Many influencers misrepresent the facts and information about certain trackers just because of endorsements or to create a 'positive' image of themselves to others. Some apps like the Nike Training Club usually do not take progressive overload into account [20]. Further, if somebody uses the same workout repeatedly or randomly selects different exercise routines each day, the results may not fully display the impact and plateau. As with any social media, another major disadvantage is that some people may get obsessed with tracking and competing, leading to stress and other adverse effects on one's physical and mental health. This has been especially seen among children who are often incentivized by virtual prizes and recognition (badges, stars, etc.). Finally, while some people willingly use fitness trackers and health apps, others just feel the pressure to keep up with the trend of using new technology in the forms of wearable trackers or apps.

In conclusion, social fitness apps, if used properly, can help people make lifestyle changes, attain health and fitness goals, and lead healthy lives. However, one must be aware of the shortcomings so that they do not impede their progress and motivation.

5.4 RESEARCH: IMPACT OF SOCIAL MEDIA ON MHEALTH

Social connections, comparisons, and recommendations have been helpful to promote fitness and the use of fitness trackers. Although generally those who are supported more by friends and family are likely to engage in increased physical activity [21], some studies have found that social support for physical activity in some cases may be more critical for those individuals who are not very active and do not exercise regularly [22]. Social support is especially important for sedentary older adults, and having an active friend often helps in bringing about positive change related to physical activity in such individuals by providing additional motivation [23].

A few research studies have focused on the impact of social media and social networking-based capabilities of fitness trackers and mHealth apps on improved health and wellness [24]. A study by Curmi et al. [25] revealed that social ties between athlete Facebook friends grew strong by sharing real-time fitness data on social media. Sharing information promotes competition, and competition stimulates increased levels of physical activity [26]. The feature of feedback to users on their overall progress and performance motivates users to become more responsible towards their health and continue to work on individual fitness goals. [27] studied the effects of integrating fitness trackers/apps data with social media networking, concerns from users about privacy, and tips for future app designs. This research was based on data from 32 users of *WeRun*, a fitness plugin in the Chinese social networking app WeChat. The 32 users included 14 females and 18 males with a diverse age group and educational background. [28] studied 55 participants to understand users' perspectives regarding an intervention based on mobile social networking to promote physical activity and discovered that the social aspect was important in enhancing engagement with the intervention technique, apart from the self-regulatory (individual) factors such as self-monitoring of behavior, goal setting, and so on. [29] conducted a meta-analysis based systematic review to understand the effect of social interaction enabled by wearable fitness tracking devices on increasing physical activity. Their research findings indicated that social interactions, such as competitions and recommendations, played a role in enhancing the physical activity of users, although they were found to act both as motivators and demotivators for individuals to engage in such activities.

5.5 CONCLUSIONS

Wearables and mobile health apps have gained popularity in the last few years, as they provide users with real-time data analysis about their health. Social media has become an integral part of human life as well. No matter the age, people these days are found scrolling through social media every few minutes on their smartphones or tablet computers. The growth of social media will continue in the future, with more advancements in technology as well as greater reliance on remote or online environments created by the recent COVID-19 pandemic and ensuing lockdowns around the world. Social media provides powerful platforms for people to develop social connections and share similar personal or career interests and activities. It is thus clear that fitness awareness among the general population has increased by the use of social media. Fitness tracker apps and wearable devices have been found helpful to some extent in changing the behavior of individuals to promote healthy living by providing timely reminders, helpful guides, and encouragement. The social media platforms and integrations have helped not only the consumers but also have provided companies with ways of marketing their products and raising awareness of brands among a much wider audience. However, as seen in this chapter, social media has both positive and negative impacts on individuals and society, so it is imperative that these are used with caution. Some challenges and concerns associated with social media applications in fitness trackers relate to the privacy and security of one's data since health and medical data are personal and sensitive and must be protected from falling into the wrong hands. Inaccurate and misleading data posted on leaderboards and shared with others can create frustration and, more importantly, affect other people's health if used as is. If used properly, social media has the capability of significantly impacting people's health and wellness via fitness trackers and mHealth apps, as we have seen in this chapter.

Although it has been established that the benefits of social networking capabilities integrated with fitness trackers outweigh the risks and concerns, more in-depth research is needed to assess their overall impact in a scientifically rigorous manner. Some studies report mixed results while some studies fail to establish anything conclusively. Studies with large sample sizes covering a diverse set of demographic distributions, strong study design (like randomized control trials), and hypotheses will lead to discoveries and results that will create confidence and trust in the minds of existing consumers so that they can continue to use these devices effectively, and they can also encourage new users to adopt them. Another aspect is that with an overwhelming amount of social media platform choices and types of electronic fitness trackers available on the market today, it can be hard to pick which social channels and trackers to use. So, research in this area to compare the functionalities, advantages, and disadvantages of various platforms and devices is also crucial to help common people make informative choices that are best suited to their needs and lifestyles.

NOTES

1 A **hashtag** – written with a # symbol – is used to index keywords or topics on Twitter. This function was created on Twitter and allows people to easily follow topics they are interested in (https://help.twitter.com).

2 **Instagram Stories** allow Instagram users to share photos and videos to their Stories – which is visible to followers of the users' Instagram accounts.

3 https://en.wikipedia.org/wiki/WeChat
4 https://en.wikipedia.org/wiki/Tencent_QQ
5 https://en.wikipedia.org/wiki/Telegram_(software)
6 www.myfitnesspal.com/
7 www.bodyspacefitness.com/
8 www.onepeloton.com/
9 www.shred.app/

REFERENCES

1. Social media Wikipedia page: https://en.wikipedia.org/wiki/Social_media, retrieved on February 27, 2019.
2. Agichtein, E., Castillo, C., Donato, D., Gionis, A., Mishne, G. (2008). Finding high-quality content in social media, *WISDOM – Proceedings of the 2008 International Conference on Web Search and Data Mining*: 183–193.
3. Kakkar, G. (2020). What are the different types of social media? *Digital Vidya blog*. Link: www.digitalvidya.com/blog/types-of-social-media/. Retrieved on August 26, 2021.
4. Foreman, C. (2017). 10 Types of social media and how each can benefit your business. *Hootsuite blog*, Link: https://blog.hootsuite.com/types-of-social-media/. Retrieved on August 26, 2021.
5. Goodrow, K. (2017). You know what's cool? A billion hours. You Tube. Link: https://blog.youtube/news-and-events/you-know-whats-cool-billion-hours/. Retrieved on August 26, 2021.
6. Metz, C. (2016). Forget Apple vs. the FBI: WhatsApp Just switched on Encryption for a Billion People. *Wired*. Archived from the original on April 5, 2016. Retrieved on August 29, 2021.
7. Amedie, J. (2015). The Impact of Social Media on Society. *Pop Culture Intersections*. 2. https://scholarcommons.scu.edu/engl_176/2. Retrieved on August 29, 2021.
8. Starr, L., Davilla, J. (2009). Excessive Discussion of Problems Between Adolescent Friends May Lead To Depression And Anxiety. *Stony Brook University*. January 27, 2009.
9. Rafla, M., Carson, N. J., Dejong, S. M. (2014). Adolescents and the Internet: What Mental Health Clinicians Need to Know, *Current Psychiatry Reports*, 16 (9): 472. doi:10.1007/s11920-014-0472-x PMID 25070673.
10. Junco, R. (2012). Too Much Face and Not Enough Books: The relationship between multiple indices of Facebook use and academic performance. *Computers in Human Behavior*. 28(1):187–198.
11. Becker, M. W., Alzahabi, R., and Hopwood, C.J. (2013). Media Multitasking Is Associated with Symptoms of Depression and Social Anxiety. *Cyberpsychology, Behavior, and Social Networking* 16(2): 132–35.

12. O'keeffe, G. S., Clarke-Pearson, K. (2011). The Impact of social media on Children, Adolescents, and Families. *Pediatrics*, 127(40): 800–804.
13. Weimann, G. (2008). The Psychology of Mass-Mediated Terrorism. *American Behavioral Scientist*, 52(1): 69–86. http://eds.a.ebscohost.com.libproxy.scu.edu/ehost/detail/
14. WebMD Wikipedia page: https://en.wikipedia.org/wiki/WebMD, retrieved of February 27, 2019.
15. Innovatemedtech (2019). Social Media in Healthcare. Link: https://innovatemedtec.com/digital-health/health-social-media-in-healthcare, retrieved on February 27, 2019.
16. Landi, H. (2016). Study: Fitbit Corporate Wellness Programs cut Employer Healthcare Costs, *Healthcare Innovation*. Link: www.hcinnovationgroup.com/population-health-management/mobile-health-mhealth/news/13027550/study-fitbit-corporate-wellness-programs-cut-employer-healthcare-costs, published on October 5, 2016. Retrieved on February 27, 2019.
17. Harris, S. (2021). The best fitness apps you can use with friends. Link: www.blissmark.com/self/best-fitness-apps-friends/. Retrieved on August 30, 2021.
18. Nguyen, A. (2021). Health and Fitness Influencers Spreading Misinformation within their Community. *Debating Communities and Networks XII*. Link: http://networkconference.netstudies.org/2021/2021/04/26/612/. Retrieved on August 31, 2021.
19. Lea Genders Fitness website (2021). A Trainer's perspective: Pros and cons of five popular fitness apps. Link: www.leagendersfitness.com/news/pros-and-cons-popular-fitness-apps, Retrieved on September 16, 2021.
20. Trost S.G., Owen N., Bauman, A.E., Sallis, J.F., Brown, W, (2002). Correlates of adults' participation in physical activity: review and update. *Medicine and Science in Sports and Exercises (MSSE)*, 34(12):1996–2001. DOI: 10.1097/00005768-200212000-00020
21. Eyler, A.A., Brownson, R.C., Donatelle, R.J., King, A.C., Brown, D., Sallis, J.F. (1999). Physical activity social support and middle- and older-aged minority women: results from a US survey. *Social Science & Medicine*, 49(6):781–9.10.1016/S0277-9536(99)00137-9.
22. King, A.C., Stokols, D., Talen, E., Brassington, G.S., Killingsworth, R. (2002). Theoretical approaches to the promotion of physical activity: forging a transdisciplinary paradigm. *American Journal of Preventive Medicine*, 23(2):15–25. DOI: 10.1016/S0749-3797(02)00470-1
23. Sullivan, A.N., & Lachman, M. E. (2017). Behavior Change with Fitness Technology in Sedentary Adults: A Review of the Evidence for Increasing Physical Activity. *Frontiers in Public Health*, 4, 289. https://doi.org/10.3389/fpubh.2016.00289.

24. Curmi, F., Ferrario, M.A., Whittle, J. (2014). Sharing real-time biometric data across social networks. In *Proceedings of the 2014 Conference on Designing Interactive Systems*, pp: 657–666, June 21–25, 2014, Vancouver, BC, Canada.
25. Shih, P.C., Han, K., Poole, E.S., Rosson, M.B., Carroll, J.M. (2015). Use and adoption challenges of wearable activity trackers. In: *Proceedings of the iConference*, March 24–27, 2015, Newport Beach, CA.
26. Gui, X., Chen, Y., Caldeira, C., Xiao, D., Chen, Y. (2017). When Fitness Meets Social Networks: Investigating Fitness Tracking and Social Practices on WeRun. In *Proceedings of the 2017 CHI Conference on Human Factors in Computing Systems*, May 2017, pp: 1647–1659. https://doi.org/10.1145/3025453.3025654.
27. Tong, H. L., Coiera, E., & Laranjo, L. (2018). Using a Mobile Social Networking App to Promote Physical Activity: A Qualitative Study of Users' Perspectives. *Journal of Medical Internet research* (JMIR), 20(12), e11439. https://doi.org/10.2196/11439.
28. Girginov, V., Moore, P., Olsen, N., Godfrey, T., Cooke, F. (2020). Wearable technology-stimulated social interaction for promoting physical activity: A systematic review. *Cogent Social Sciences*, 6(1), DOI: 10.1080/23311886.2020.1742517

CHAPTER 6

Issues and Challenges in mHealth Technology

6.1 INTRODUCTION

As with any technology, mobile healthcare is not without its issues and challenges. Despite reports of the potential explosive growth of this industry over the next few years, one must pay attention to the various concerns, issues, and challenges that this technology faces today. That is only how the technology, which has huge potential for improving how people perceive and approach healthcare and individual health management today, will actually lead to positive impact on health outcomes of the society via wider adoption and acceptability. Such challenges cover a broad range, from privacy and security concerns related to the data collected by fitness tracking devices and mobile health apps, to the nature of the data collected to organizational policies, regulations, and support. All these are major aspects of mHealth technology but are different and hence must be addressed individually and adequately.

In this chapter, we discuss some of these primary challenges facing the mHealth technology and offer some potential solutions. Section 6.2 thus outlines these various issues, Section 6.3 presents some potential solutions, and we finally conclude in Section 6.4.

DOI: 10.1201/9780429428449-6

6.2 ISSUES AND CHALLENGES OF MHEALTH TECHNOLOGY

We focus on six different types of issues and challenges underlying the mobile healthcare technology in this chapter – namely, (i) privacy and security concerns, (ii) organizational and regulatory policies and support, (iii) sustaining consumer use and behavior, (iv) reliability and accuracy of data, (v) lack of rigorous research findings, and (vi) design, affordability, and other usability issues. This is not meant to be an exhaustive list of all issues since this is an evolving technology that continues to expand in new directions, along with which come new barriers and challenges.

6.2.1 Privacy and Security Concerns

Fitness trackers and mobile apps capture massive amounts of data from users. This includes personal data that are typically entered by the user, such as birth date, weight, height, photos, links to social media networking sites and list of friends, and so on. Further, the tracker and app also collect health or biometric data that include the number of daily steps taken, number of daily minutes doing more rigorous exercises (referred to as 'active minutes'), distance traveled, etc. Health indicators such as heart rate, skin temperature, blood oxygenation levels, etc., are also recorded by most advanced fitness trackers and apps. Finally, mobile apps are used by healthcare professionals to collect more detailed health-related data like blood pressure, blood sugar levels, ECG, and information on medications, clinical diagnosis, and treatment plans for patients. Metadata from these trackers, such as GPS coordinates, timestamps for different activities, and unique usernames, etc., are also continually recorded.

Apart from the fact that health information and other data collected by fitness trackers are of a personal and sensitive nature, the most concerning fact is that when such large quantities of data collected constantly over a period time are combined with other data, one can easily determine the identity of an individual and their behaviors. Hence if the systems that collect and store these types of data are breached or hacked, this can lead to serious losses of confidential information, which can cause potential harm if falling in the hands of criminals. Such harmful effects include privacy violations, financial losses, losses of intellectual property, and losses of other personal and professional data. However, fitness tracker users are often unaware of the privacy implications and resulting consequences of how the data could be misused, and therefore knowledge about data losses becomes known only after the fact – in most cases, when much damage has already been inflicted.

Then there are the security concerns of mobile devices themselves. It is much easier for a doctor to misplace or lose a smartphone than it is a stack of files or a computer. These devices are also more likely to be targeted by thieves. If they happen to store patient information locally on their phones or try to access a database or patient portal remotely, anyone with access suddenly has a trove of personal information at their disposal. Some organizations also have now chosen to adopt a bring-your-own-device (BYOD) policy that allows doctors, nurses, and other employees to use their own personal mobile phones and tablet computers to use for work-related tasks, which exposes them to additional security concerns, as individual devices usually do not have the same high level of security provided by company IT. Similarly, individuals can lose their smartphones (either misplaced or stolen) that record their health and fitness data. If those mobile devices are not protected via strong passwords or biometrics (like fingerprints or FaceID in iPhones), data stored in them can be easily accessed and misused by thieves.

There are also legitimate concerns about the security of citizen information by programs using mobile health technologies. In particular, message transmission security and data storage security can put citizen information at risk if the necessary precautions with respect to protection and safeguarding are not taken. Many recent events highlight potential risks. In 2018, Strava uploaded a heat map of users' anonymous and aggregate fitness tracking data on their website that revealed the locations and behaviors of military personnel using such fitness apps at certain secret military bases in Afghanistan, Iraq, and Syria [1]. During that same year, fitness tracker accounts of 150 million MyFitnessPal users were hacked by unauthorized users who gained access to names, usernames, and passwords of account holders of that app [2]. As a result of this significant data breach, personal identifying information of these millions of people was compromised, which could potentially have led to more serious consequences such as fraud, identity theft, and even financial losses. A recent news item [3] reported that fitness data tracked and shared by employer-sponsored wellness programs can have consequences. An employee may not be aware of the fact that their employer is able to track their physical activity without their knowledge. For example, a certain employer commented on an employee's increased physical activity who later suffered a heart attack. Although this was not considered intrusive and maybe beneficial to an extent (if medical attention was obtained quickly as a result of the employer's intervention), this incident did raise privacy concerns regarding how much of personal fitness and health data of employees should be accessible to employers. Further, some insurance companies have also been known to track their customers' exercise and health data, along with eating habits [4]. Although often perceived as beneficial when they award incentives and rewards to their members for leading healthy lives, people have been concerned that such monitoring can also lead to increased premiums in the future based on certain symptoms and health data indicators.

6.2.2 Organizational, Regulatory, and Support

It is a known fact that the healthcare industry is one of the most regulated industries today, and hence the mHealth space today faces unique regulatory hurdles. mHealth companies need to be aware of and take into account the different health-related laws that are in effect in different states across the United States that include payment, medical board requirements, and prescription regulations [5]. In many states, mHealth services can only be used with a patient after a one-on-one consultation has occurred with the doctor. Additionally, there are federal laws and regulations in place to protect the privacy and security of an individual's personal health data. One example of such a regulation is the *Health Insurance Portability and Accountability Act (HIPAA)* introduced by the Office of Civil Rights under the Department of Health and Human Services (HHS) in 1996, which for the first time introduced national standards for protecting every person's health information, including those stored in an electronic format [6]. The underlying rules of this act require authorization from the individual involved to share or access their health data while preserving the right to request and obtain their own health information. Since then, the act has evolved, and new sets of security regulations have been instituted that include administrative, technical, and physical safeguards for protected

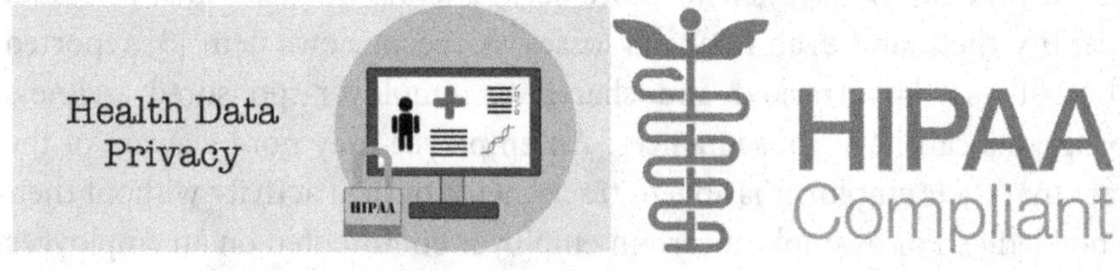

FIGURE 6.1 HIPAA. (Creative Commons License.)[1,2]

health information, such as that collected by healthcare providers, hospitals and clinics, insurance companies, and even companies that design and maintain electronic health records (EHRs) [7].

Hence, in order to use mobile devices and physical fitness tracking devices for managing individual health and well-being, all these regulations are needed to be met, and the companies who develop these technologies need to be aware of what federal and state-level organizations (like the FDA and HSS, for example) will have the oversight of the products they develop so that they can keep abreast of all the new rules and regulations that come into effect.

Another issue facing mobile healthcare technology is the availability of the appropriate support at the backend so that mobile devices can continue to function properly. A strong and consistent wireless signal is the minimum requirement for networks to provide service throughout its network for mHealth services to work seamlessly and effectively. At the same time, these networks need to be equipped with adequate security protocols to protect the privacy of the health and fitness data that are collected and transmitted by the various devices and apps that are using that network. The availability of IT trained IT personnel is extremely important to provide support when necessary and ensure that problems are resolved as quickly as possible. This issue can pose considerable challenges to small clinics and healthcare companies that may not necessarily have the resources to hire and maintain a skilled tech team.

6.2.3 Reliability and Accuracy of Data

Some fitness tracking devices, both wearables and mobile apps, have been found to have some inaccuracies while reporting data measurements. Several research studies have been conducted to understand how accurate the measurements collected by mHealth devices are and were discussed at length in Chapter 4. Despite some studies reporting that mHealth devices are fairly accurate [8], many others have demonstrated that popularly used fitness trackers (like Fitbits) are less accurate in measuring steps, tracking distances covered, and recording calories burned during physical activities in certain scenarios [9]. Some other advanced fitness trackers have been found to have inaccuracies in heart-rate monitoring [10]. In fact, [11] observed that although the common fitness trackers like Fitbit, Apple Watch, and Samsung were able to measure steps more or less accurately, heart-rate measurements were quite variable, particularly for Fitbit trackers, while Apple Watch and Garmin trackers were slightly better in terms of accuracy. Further reports [12] have shown that some readily available low-cost apps are not based on research evidence, which tend to produce incorrect information that can potentially mislead users. Unreliability in this instance is more evident when the application has not been reviewed and approved by a regulatory organization like the U.S. Food and Drug Administration (FDA).

All of the above facts and findings can make users hesitant to trust the data collected by mHealth devices and hence can deter both consistent usage and widespread adoption. More importantly, lack of data accuracy and information integrity in mHealth technology can cause harm to patients and prevent efficient health management. This can potentially limit the benefits of such promising technology to a considerable extent.

6.2.4 Lack of Rigorous Research and Findings

As discussed already in Chapter 4, scientific research on fitness trackers is limited, and research findings are often inconclusive or misleading. Some studies have indeed reported positive impacts of wearable devices or mobile apps on users' health and health goals [13], whereas others have failed to observe any such impact at all [14]. In fact, [15] found that for the group of people who were provided a fitness tracker ('intervention' group in a randomized control study setup) actually lost less weight compared to the other 'control' group who did not use a tracking device, and similarly, a randomized controlled trial involving 800 subjects found that after one year of use, a fitness tracker had no effect on the subjects' overall health and

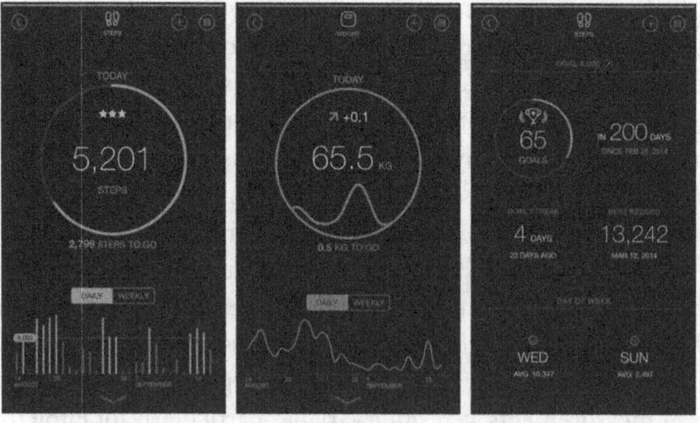

FIGURE 6.2 Fitness tracker data and findings. (Creative Commons License.)[3]

fitness, despite the offer of financial incentives [16]. Chapter 4 contains a detailed overview of existing research on mHealth apps and devices.

A large portion of the population worldwide trusts science and hence develops confidence in new technology based on positive outcomes reported by rigorous scientific studies. Judging by that, the lack of consistent promising results for mHealth apps and devices may act as a potential deterrent to more widespread adoption of this technology. Moreover, current users may lose motivation in the continued usage of their devices once they learn about such research studies that do not show positive benefits of using these devices.

6.2.5 Design, Affordability, User Interface, and Other Usability Considerations

Usability plays a critical role in driving consumer decisions to adopt and use any technology device. The case for mHealth technology is no different. In addition to privacy and security concerns and those related to the reliability and validity of the data collected by these studies, additional research has shown that the comfort level of these wearable fitness products is the key to its success in terms of acceptance among ordinary consumers; product usability is an important aspect of this [17, 18].

Some studies have reported that individuals have stopped using wearables only a few months after purchase because the devices were not comfortable to wear on a regular basis, and some have mentioned that the process of tracking activities is cumbersome and confusing [19]. Others have stated that the primary reason for not using a wearable fitness device is the cost, as most of the advanced trackers cost hundreds of dollars. Apart from that, many people, mostly older adults and people belonging to developing countries, are not always as familiar with technology. So, although they may use smartphones, tracking fitness data and managing their health on such devices may prove to be a cumbersome task. For instance, many users are known not to sync their physical tracker with their mobile device on a regular basis, thus failing to monitor their daily physical activities. Moreover, the process of taking ECG measurements or measuring blood oxygen levels is complex for most of the physical devices (like Apple Watches). This can prevent many people from leveraging these advanced functionalities of mHealth devices to the fullest for effective self-health management, the primary purpose of this technology. Similarly, many kids use these fitness trackers today (Fitbit Ace, for instance), so these devices should be navigable by these young users as well.

6.2.6 Sustaining Consumer Use and Behavior

Although many individuals are using mHealth devices today, primarily the wearable trackers, there are concerns regarding sustaining that use among consumers. Although such devices can be effective in motivating people to be healthier and active, many consumers are abandoning them soon after purchase [20]. In one recent research study, 40% of the people stopped wearing the fitness tracking device within the first six months, despite cash incentives provided by researchers to the participants in the study [21]. Yet the proliferation of wearable technologies coincides with a worldwide issue of obesity and poor health. In the United States, 80% of adults do not meet the government's national recommendations for aerobic activity and muscle strengthening [hhs.gov]. Thus, one may wonder: How does this happen during a time when wearable technology consumption continues to grow and become mainstream?

The major driver of sustained use is self-motivation, and there are a number of factors that affect motivation in a person. Some of these may include lack of proper knowledge about how to use the mHealth devices properly, how to interpret the data that they display, and underlying concerns regarding privacy, security and confidentiality, technology issues, and cost.

6.3 POTENTIAL SOLUTIONS TO ISSUES AND CHALLENGES

The overall goal of effective security protocols is to protect participant identity and secure data in such a way that if unauthorized individuals were to gain access, they would be unable to link the data with a particular person or with other data being sent.

6.3.1 Security and Privacy Issues

The common ways in which companies ensure security are by providing encryption mechanisms on data traversal to and from server and device, requiring users to authenticate every time they want to access the information or device, and providing privacy policies that contain detailed information about what data are collected and how they are being stored and used. For example, enabling WPA2 encryption on mobile devices enhances the security of data and information transmitted over wireless networks by preserving the anonymity of the users. Even simpler techniques such as setting a strong password (consisting of different letters, numbers, and special characters like !, %,*, etc.) or a strong personal identification number or PIN (six to eight digits instead of the usual four) can be exercised by the general people to add some layer of protection on personal devices. Adequate training and support in this regard about how to set effective passwords or PINs (for example, not to use the word 'password' or simple phrases like 'abcd' as passwords or use '1234' or birthday as PINs) are very important in this respect, especially for older adults and young kids who may not have the requisite technology literacy to fully understand the risks associated with weaker security measures on their personal mobile devices.

Once the data are encrypted and protected, Virtual Private Networks (VPNs) can also be employed to securely transmitting the data collected by mHealth devices and apps to the servers that are meant for processing and analyzing them. VPNs have been known to be used quite widely in mHealth communities already [22]. Sometimes the use of a VPN on a mobile device may be challenging and can slow down the system and hence may not be as commonly used by the general population. In addition to VPNs, various mechanisms can be applied to protect data in transit [6]. For example, data can be transferred in different orientations for further protection and in an efficient way so as to prevent the systems from becoming overwhelmed. Moreover, consumers should be more aware of security risks and follow stronger security protocols when using public networks and public devices, as those are not as safe their home or work environments and hence are more vulnerable to data breaches.

6.3.1.1 Stronger Security via Biometrics

mHealth companies can also consider employing alternative encryption and protection measures that are stronger and can enhance the level of security of these devices beyond their current levels, such as *biometrics*. Biometrics denote unique physical and behavioral characteristics of an individual that can be used for identification or authentication. Biometrics have been successfully deployed in several applications, such as law enforcement, immigration and border control, finance, and education to add extra layers of security and protection and have also made their ways into healthcare. Some application areas within the healthcare industry where biometrics such as fingerprint scans and facial images are slowly being adopted include electronic health records (EHRs) and other sensitive patient information, scheduling appointments with doctors and clinics, and physical access control for hospital staff, etc. Not only do biometrics provide better security and act as better identifiers than a patient's demographic data, but they also help in reducing medical errors and streamline data sharing protocols. Thus, given the promise of this technology to make the entire healthcare delivery process more efficient, its foray into mHealth is imminent. No progress has yet been made in this regard, but the use of biometrics in telemedicine has already started. A Canadian healthcare technology company recently explored using biometric-enabled mobile drug dispensaries. These in-home devices use facial recognition to dispense drugs and record that the prescription was taken as recommended [23].

Multimodal biometrics, or biometric technology that is based on fusion of information from more than one biometric trait (such as face + fingerprints, fingerprints + iris), are also becoming popular now, which can grant even more security to data and devices than traditional unimodal biometric systems based on a single biometric trait. This is because although single biometric traits have been compromised with advances in technology, it becomes increasingly more difficult to steal or spoof multiple physical traits of an individual. Therefore, they offer additional security that is essential for healthcare services, and for this reason, research resources should be devoted to developing multimodal biometrics for mHealth devices and applications to keep confidential and sensitive health data protected with the utmost security measures.

Lastly, it must be mentioned that even in a perfect world, no system involving humans can be expected to be completely secure. As technology continues to evolve at a rapid pace, more and more sophisticated approaches to hacking will continue to appear, leading to data breaches. Thus, a balance must be established between security, subject usability, and available resources to meet the requirements of the particular mHealth technology. The main objective should thus be to mitigate security risks

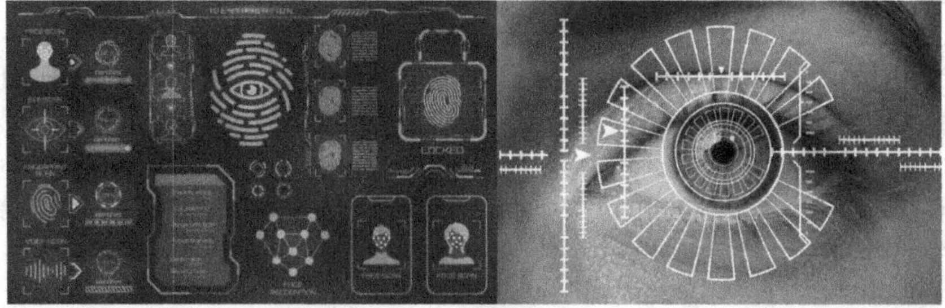

FIGURE 6.3 Some examples of biometric traits used commonly in identification and authentication applications. (Creative Commons License.)[4,5]

as much as possible without impeding use, while at the same time to have strong safeguards to protect against personal data losses.

6.3.2 Effective Policy Making

Effective policy will become increasingly important as the field of mHealth matures. Data security is a particularly important issue to address within the area of policy. Policy makers and program managers need to be made aware of security issues in the mHealth domain so appropriate policies and strategies can be developed and implemented. Policies will also be vital to efforts in harmonizing eHealth and mHealth initiatives and directions in the short- and long-term. There are several laws and regulations that all mHealth companies need to adhere to, such as HIPAA; GDPR (General Data Protection Regulation) which is a law in the European Union that deals with the collection, storage, sharing, or transfer of data for European users; FDA clearance; HL7 (a mHealth work group that develops and promotes technology standards and frameworks for mHealth), and so on [24, 25], so it is critical for those companies to share these policies, along with their own policies regarding data collection, storage, and analysis with their users at the very beginning. Transparency in this respect thus plays an important role in educating users as well as ensuring that there is no misunderstanding on their part that may deter wider acceptability.

Many policies and measures may also depend on the location and may apply to sub-groups of the population. For instance, the latest regulation is the U.S. California Consumer Privacy Act (CCPA), which provides consumers in California with more transparency on how their personal data are being utilized. The consumers have the right to know what data are collected, where they are stored, to whom they are sold, and the right to disclosure. Similarly, COPPA (Children's Online Privacy Protection Act) is a U.S. act that prohibits online services and companies to use or collect children's data (below 13 years) without permissions from their parents or guardians. It is not possible for people to know about all of these different policies and regulations, so it is again the responsibility of the mHealth companies to make their consumers aware of these with full transparency.

6.3.3 Rigorous Research and Evaluation Techniques

MHealth companies should devote additional resources into testing and evaluation of their health and fitness products (both apps and physical trackers) in order to ensure more accurate and reliable measurements and data collection. The better the quality of data gathered and analyzed, the more trust and confidence users will have in them, and that will in turn motivate them to keep using these products if they are already users and even encourage new users to adopt them for their potential benefits. Moreover, evaluation techniques are necessary to improve the security underlying mHealth technology (as discussed above) as well as to improve user experience and user acceptance (as discussed below).

6.3.4 Other Issues

According to International Organization for Standardization [26], the usability of a specific product includes three aspects – namely, effectiveness, efficiency, and satisfaction rating. Usability tests and evaluations aim to make medical equipment easier, safer, and more effective and pleasant for users. This is thus a critical component that designers of mHealth must focus on because a usability evaluation helps wearable devices to satisfy the requirements of the market and consumers [27]. Such evaluation techniques and the consequent improvements will help the increase acceptability and adoption of this technology rapidly among the wider population. Research studies in this area of user acceptance and user experience can also be considerably expanded since not too many of them exist currently [28,29]. Further, the costs of these products can be decreased also for more affordability among the general population.

6.4 CONCLUSIONS

According to World Health Organization (WHO), mHealth can transform the delivery of health services across the globe and bring about a paradigm shift in healthcare delivery processes [30]. This is propelled by huge advances in wireless and mobile technology and applications, computing and storage capabilities (like cloud services), and the increasing number of smartphone users all over the world. However, this growth of mHealth technology will not be able to continue smoothly if the various issues and challenges outlined in this chapter are not thoroughly investigated, analyzed, and addressed. As companies focus on designing and developing newer and newer mHealth applications, services, and devices, it is equally important for them to devote a substantial number of resources to understanding and addressing these challenges. Although we have offered some potential solutions to these challenges, it is quite apparent that not all of these will be resolved once and for all and very easily, but the requisite work and efforts should be ongoing at a rapid pace. As technology continues its exponential growth in the next decade or so, newer challenges are also likely to emerge, and all companies and organizations involved in mHealth technology should be sufficiently prepared to adapt quickly and address those sooner rather than later.

NOTES

1 https://i1.wp.com/sitn.hms.harvard.edu/wp-content/uploads/2019/05/Cover_Harrod.png?resize=1911%2C763
2 https://technofaq.org/wp-content/uploads/2017/11/hipaa-compliant-logo-620x350.png
3 http://1.bp.blogspot.com/-PalW7Vk5U8k/VCWdjOxAq_I/AAAAAAAALJQ/U4sLZMvNyKE/s1600/APple.png
4 https://nedhayes.com/wp-content/uploads/2020/06/GettyImages-957612422-660x396.jpg
5 https://cdn.pixabay.com/photo/2017/09/21/08/56/eye-2771174_960_720.jpg

REFERENCES

1. Perez-Pena, R. and Rosenberg, M. (2018). Strava fitness app can reveal military sites, analysts say. *New York Times*, published on January 29, 2018. Link: www.nytimes.com/2018/01/29/world/middleeast/strava-heat-map.html. Retrieved on November 1, 2021.
2. Shaban, H. (2018). Under Armor announces data breach, affecting 150 million MyFitnessPal app accounts, *The Washington Post*, published on March 29, 2018. Link: www.washingtonpost.com/news/the-switch/wp/2018/03/29/under-armour-announces-data-breach-affecting-150-million-myfitnesspal-app-accounts/. Retrieved on November 1, 2021.
3. Rowland, C. (2019). With fitness trackers in the workplace, bosses can monitor your every step – and possibly more, *The Washington Post*, published on February 16, 2019. Link: www.washingtonpost.com/business/economy/with-fitness-trackers-in-the-workplace-bosses-can-monitor-your-every-step--and-possibly-more/2019/02/15/75ee0848-2a45-11e9-b011-d8500644dc98_story.html. Retrieved on November 2, 2021.
4. Marr, B. (2019). This health insurance company tracks customers' exercise and eating habits using big data and IoT, *Forbes*, published on March 27, 2019. Link: www.forbes.com/sites/bernardmarr/2019/05/27/this-health-insurance-company-tracks-customers-exercise-and-eating-habits-using-big-data-and-iot/?sh=7c850f686ef3. Retrieved on November 2, 2021.

5. Mcaskill, R. (2015). The Challenges of implementing mHealth, *mHealth Intelligence*, link: https://mhealthintelligence.com/news/the-challenges-of-implementing-mhealth, published on February 9, 2015. Retrieved on February 27, 2019.
6. Arora, S., Yttri, J., & Nilse, W. (2014). Privacy and Security in Mobile Health (mHealth) Research. *Alcohol Research: current reviews*, 36(1), 143–151.
7. U.S. Department of Health and Human Services (2013). Modifications to the HIPAA Privacy, Security, Enforcement, and Breach Notification Rules Under the Health Information Technology for Economic and Clinical Health Act and the Genetic Information Nondiscrimination Act, 2013. Link: www.federalregister.gov/documents/2013/01/25/2013-01073/modifications-to-the-hipaa-privacy-security-enforcement-and-breach-notification-rules-under-the. Retrieved on October 16, 2021.
8. Ricchio, K., Lyter, P., Palao, J. M. (2018). Reliability of fitness trackers at different prices for measuring steps and heart rate: a pilot study. *Central European Journal of Sport Sciences and Medicine*, 24: 57–64.
9. Feehan, L. M., Geldman, J., Sayre, E. C., Park, C., Ezzat, A. M., Yoo, J. Y., Hamilton, C. B., & Li, L. C. (2018). Accuracy of Fitbit Devices: Systematic Review and Narrative Syntheses of Quantitative Data, *Journal of Medical Internet Research* (JMIR); mHealth and uHealth, 6(8), e10527. Doi: https://doi.org/10.2196/10527.
10. Kroll, R.R., Boyd, J.G., Maslove, D.M. (2016). Accuracy of a Wrist-Worn Wearable Device for Monitoring Heart Rates in Hospital Inpatients: A Prospective Observational Study, *Journal of Medical Internet Research* (JMIR);18(9):e253. doi: 10.2196/jmir.6025
11. Fuller, D., Colwell, E., Low, J., Orychock, K., Tobin, M.A., Simango, B., Buote, R., Van Heerden, D., Luan, H., Cullen, K., Slade, L., Taylor, N.G.A. (2020). Reliability and Validity of Commercially Available Wearable Devices for Measuring Steps, Energy Expenditure, and Heart Rate: Systematic Review, *Journal of Medical Internet Research (JMIR) Mhealth Uhealth* 2020; 8(9): e18694. doi: https://mhealth.jmir.org/2020/9/e18694/.
12. Scher, D.L. (2015). The Big Problem with Mobile Health Apps. *Medscape*. Link: www.medscape. com/viewarticle/840335. Retrieved on November 1, 2021.
13. Stiglbauer, B., Weber, S., Batinic, B. (2019). Does your health really benefit from using a self-tracking device? Evidence from a longitudinal randomized control trial. *Computers in Human Behavior*, 94, 131–139.
14. Schaben, J.A., Furness, S. (2018). Investing in college students: the role of fitness tracker. *Digital Health*, 2018 Apr 4, 4: 2055207618766800. DOI: 10.1177/2055207618766800
15. Jakicic, J.M., Davis, K.K., Rogers, R.J., et al (2016). Effect of Wearable Technology Combined with a Lifestyle Intervention on Long-term Weight

Loss: The IDEA Randomized Clinical Trial. Journal of the American Medical Association (JAMA), 316(11): 1161–1171.

16. Finkelstein, E.A., Haaland, B.A., Bilger, M., et al. (2016). Effectiveness of activity trackers with and without incentives to increase physical activity (TRIPPA): a randomized controlled trial. The Lancet: Diabetes & Endocrinology, 4(12): 983–995.
17. Wen, D., Zhang, X., Lei, J. (2017). Consumers' perceived attitudes to wearable devices in health monitoring in China: a survey study. *Computational Methods and Programs in Biomedicine,* 140: 131–137. DOI: 10.1016/j.cmpb.2016.12.009
18. Mercer, K., Giangregorio, L., Schneider, E., Chilana, P., Li, M., Grindrod, K. (2016). Acceptance of commercially available wearable activity trackers among adults aged over 50 and with chronic illness: a mixed-methods evaluation. *Journal of Medical Internet Research (JMIR) Mhealth Uhealth,* 27; 4(1):e7. DOI: 10.2196/mhealth.4225
19. Liang, J., Xian, D., Liu, X., Fu, J., Zhang, X., Tang, B., & Lei, J. (2018). Usability Study of Mainstream Wearable Fitness Devices: Feature Analysis and System Usability Scale Evaluation. . *Journal of Medical Internet Research (JMIR) mHealth and uHealth,* 6(11), e11066. https://doi.org/10.2196/11066.
20. Rupp, M.A., Michaelis, J.R., McConnell, D.S., and Smither, J.A. (2018). The Role of Individual Differences on Perceptions of Wearable Fitness Device Trust, Usability, and Motivational Impact, *Applied Ergonomics,* 70: 77–87.
21. U.S. Department of Health and Human Services. Healthy People 2010. Available at: www.cdc.gov/nchs/healthy_people/hp2010.htm, retrieved on March 27, 2019.
22. Adibi, S., Wickramasinghe, N., Chan, C (2013). The cloud computing paradigm for mobile health. *International Journal of Soft Computing and Software Engineering* 3(3): 403–410.
23. Aware blog (2021). Biometrics in healthcare: Improved safety and privacy for patients. Link: www.aware.com/blog-biometrics-in-healthcare/. Retrieved on November 7, 2021.
24. Nurgaliev, L., O'Callaghan, D., Doherty, G. (2020). Security and Privacy of mHealth Applications: A Scoping Review, IEEE Access, 8: 104247-104268, 2020, DOI: 10.1109/ACCESS.2020.2999934
25. Sampat, B. H., Prabhakar, B. (2017) Privacy Risks and Security Threats in mHealth apps, *Journal of International Technology and Information Management,* 26(4), Article 5. Retrieved from https://scholarworks.lib.csusb.edu/jitim/vol26/iss4/5
26. Usability Partners (1998). ISO Standards in usability and user-centered design – ISO 9241-11 (1998) guidance in usability Link: www.usabilitypartners.se/about-usability/iso-standards website. Retrieved on November 15, 2021.

27. Yan, Y., Wang, G., Liu, S., Wu, H., Zhang, Q. (2012). Usability evaluation of infusion pump based on system usability scale. *China Medical Devices*, 10(1): 25–27.
28. McCallum, C., Rooksby, J., Gray, C.M. (2018). Evaluating the impact of physical activity apps and wearables: interdisciplinary review. *Journal of Medical Internet Research (JMIR) Mhealth Uhealth*, 6(3): e58. doi: 10.2196/mhealth.9054. http://mhealth.jmir.org/2018/3/e58/
29. Schenkenfelder, R., Selinger, S. (2018). A Comparison of Multiple Wearable Devices Regarding their User Experience During Running. Link: http://ffhoarep.fh-ooe.at/bitstream/123456789/686/1/125_218_Schenkenfelder_FullPaper_en_Final.pdf. Retrieved on November 15, 2021.
30. World Health Organization. mHealth: New horizons for health through mobile technologies. Available online, link: www.who.int/goe/publications/goe_mhealth_web.pdf. Retrieved on October 4, 2021.

CHAPTER 7

The Road Ahead for mHealth

7.1 INTRODUCTION

This entire book has shown how the technology of mobile healthcare (or mHealth) has evolved and grown over the past decade or so and has become one of the most impactful healthcare tools of the century so far. Leveraging the power of technology and penetration of smartphones, it has revolutionized the way people think about self-health and wellness management. Starting with the simple pedometer that originated in the 18th century, which was meant to count the number of steps walked and distance covered while walking, wearable fitness devices like the Apple Watch are now equipped with advanced functionalities to monitor heart rates and skin temperature, measure ECG and blood oxygenation levels, and even record dietary intake, sleep patterns, and additional exercise and workout activities performed by the user. Mobile health, or mHealth, apps, on the other hand, have also diversified considerably and have provided users with access to critical health and medical information, ability to monitor symptoms and obtain assistance in conducting clinical diagnosis, manage chronic health conditions, set up health alerts and schedule doctor appointments, manage health insurance activities, and maintain healthy living. In the era of the COVID-19 pandemic since March 2020, several apps have been launched for remotely tracking patient symptoms and performing diagnosis, scheduling, and managing vaccination appointments, among other things. The latter clearly shows how easy it has become for providers (like businesses

DOI: 10.1201/9780429428449-7

and governments) to quickly develop such technology as the need arises that has massive outreach within a very short timeframe. Consumers also benefit from such easy-to-use technology platforms that can be easily downloaded and installed on mobile devices (usually for free).

In this concluding chapter of the book, we discuss the future of mHealth technology briefly in Section 7.2 (some of which we have discussed in previous chapters as well), summarize the main challenges that pose barriers to more widespread adoption on mHealth technology in Section 7.3, and finally present a few case studies and use cases in Section 7.4, which is expected to provide the reader with a broader understanding of the capabilities and outreach of mobile healthcare technology and generate ideas for the development of more novel and innovative applications in the future. We conclude with a brief overview some potential areas of growth in mHealth technology in Section 7.5.

7.2 THE FUTURE OF MHEALTH

It is not difficult to visualize that this technology field will continue to grow and improve health outcomes significantly for the population at large. According to a report published in February 2021 [1], the global mHealth market was valued at $45.7 billion dollars and is expected to grow at a compound annual growth rate (CAGR) of 17.6% from 2021 to 2028. This is driven by the rising demand for preventive healthcare and the awareness among the general public of the need to stay active and fit. Furthermore, government initiatives have led to widescale adoption of both mobile apps and wearable devices by patients, medical professionals, healthcare providers, and other stakeholders (like insurance companies, for example). Figure 7.1 below shows the market trend in mHealth technology over the next few years. With increasing levels of internet connectivity, the power of mobile computing and smart devices, more and more mobile apps and wearables will flood the market in the years to come.

This utilization of mHealth technology increased even more significantly during the COVID-19 pandemic-driven lockdown, when access to doctors, hospitals, and gyms was severely restricted – according to data available, the number of medical apps downloaded at that time showed a spike of 65% at the global level. Apart from the usual monitoring and tracking, mHealth technologies have also played a big role in mitigating response efforts for the pandemic across the globe [2]. For instance, some nations have developed quarantine apps to enforce quarantine measures

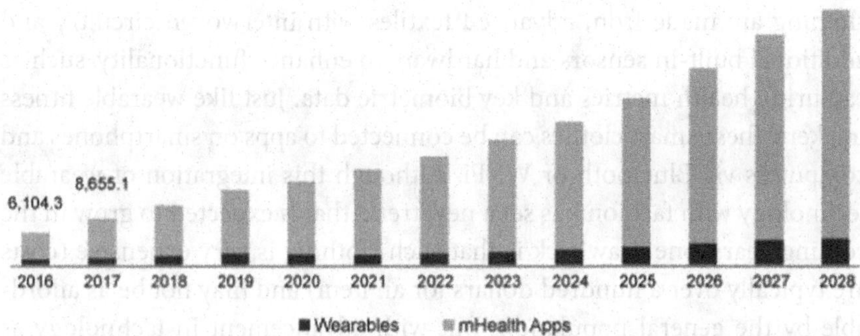

FIGURE 7.1 U.S. market size for both mobile apps and wearable devices from 2016 to 2028. (Source: Grandview Research: www.grandviewresearch.com/industry-analysis/mhealth-market.)

and apps to monitor medical professionals for COVID-19 symptoms in hospitals and clinics. Hence, in the cases of future pandemics, we are confident that this technology can prove to be a valuable tool and contribute significantly to its mitigation and control.

7.2.1 New Wearable Devices

Although in this book we have mainly focused on wearable devices on the wrist, arm, or waist, new forms of wearables are also appearing in the market and leading us towards a better-connected lifestyle. These include *wearable clothing* and *wearable jewelry* that come equipped with functional technology.

The consumer wearable clothing industry is relatively new – there are smart shirts for athletes that are fitted with GPS, accelerometers, and biomedical sensors for health and fitness monitoring; there are smart jackets that can automatically cool or warm the body based on body temperature recorded regularly by sensors embedded in the jacket itself. Among some of the more well-known brands experimenting with smart clothing are Under Armour, Levi's, Tommy Hilfiger, Samsung, Ralph Lauren, and Google [3]. One example is Ralph Lauren's *PoloTech* t-shirts,[1] which can be connected to a smartphone app to record fitness activity and track heart rate, breathing, and calories burned, as well as recommend new workouts to the wearer. Smart socks and in-shoe sensors are also available, which are used for tracking and analyzing the users' motion as they walk or run. For instance, Sensoria's smart socks[2] can detect which part of one's feet are receiving the most pressure during a run. All of these kinds of smart clothing are made from advanced textiles with interwoven circuitry and additional built-in sensors and hardware to enhance functionality, such as capturing health metrics and key biometric data. Just like wearable fitness trackers, these smart clothes can be connected to apps on smartphones and computers via Bluetooth or Wi-Fi. Although this integration of wearable technology with fashion has set a new trend that is expected to grow in the coming years, one drawback is that such clothing is very expensive (costs are typically over a hundred dollars for an item) and may not be as affordable by the general population. But with advancement in technology as newer and newer models are developed, costs may eventually go down and lead to more widespread adoption.

Among smart jewelry, rings, bracelets, and necklaces are available in the market today, which offer several features, such as fitness tracking, notifications, alarms, and even mindfulness reminders [4]. Some examples include the *Oura* smart ring, which has a built-in heart-rate monitor and can track sleep and body temperature, and *Bellabeat's Leaf Urban* that can be worn as a bracelet or a necklace or as a brooch and can track physical activity (active minutes, calories burned, distance traveled), stress level, mindfulness, and sleep. Besides, there are smartwatches that look like

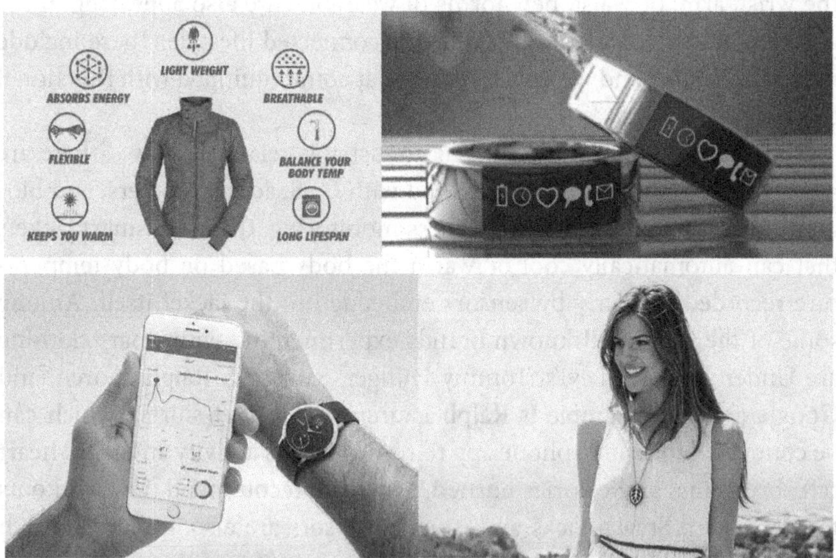

FIGURE 7.2 Examples of smart clothing and smart jewelry (License: CC.)

Note: Top left: smart jacket, top right: Oura ring, Bottom left: Withings smartwatch, Bottom right: Bellabeat's Urban Leaf worn as a necklace.

'normal' watch accessories with leather or metal bands but have embedded smart features, like the Withings Steel HR (has a heart-rate monitor and can track fitness activity) and Fossil's Carlie (can track physical activity). As with smart clothing, these smart jewelry items also come with associated mobile apps that can be utilized by users to visualize tracked activity, health, and biometric data in an easy-to-understand format. Figure 7.2 shows some currently available smart clothing and jewelry.

The future for such mHealth technology is very bright, and vast opportunities exist to create new and more advanced mobile apps and wearables of various kinds. However, in order to sustain its growth and expansion, one needs to keep in mind the underlying issues and challenges and address them adequately for greater proliferation and adoption across different population groups. We discuss these in the next section.

7.3 ADDRESSING CHALLENGES AND IMPROVING ACCEPTABILITY

The main issues and challenges facing mobile healthcare technology today were discussed in depth in Chapter 6, along with potential solutions. We briefly summarize some of these major challenges in this section since these are of the utmost importance in order for the positive impacts of mHealth technology to spread more widely.

Overall, we identified six major components of challenges in implementing mHealth: (i) privacy and security concerns, (ii) organizational and regulatory policies and support, (iii) sustaining consumer use and behavior, (iv) reliability and accuracy of data, (v) lack of rigorous research findings, and (vi) design, affordability, and other usability issues. Some potential solutions to these challenges to mHealth would include stronger encryption and protection mechanisms, such as those provided by biometrics (like face, fingerprints, iris) to safeguard personal data; more rigorous and large-scale research studies to assess potential benefits of this technology; accuracy, reliability, and usability issues; and more effective policy making and user training to create awareness of the different rules and regulations that govern the use of different mHealth devices and apps and the data collected and used from them. Further, designing more affordable and reliable physical trackers that will be comfortable to wear will also go a long way in making them more acceptable and popular among the general population. For instance, fitness trackers specifically designed for kids (such as the Fitbit Ace) should be simple to use and have an attractive look and features for children to start using them more to track their health and physical activities on a regular basis.

mHealth is surely a much-needed boon for improving the healthcare delivery process today and for the personal health and wellness management of individual consumers. However, these challenges call for a focus on areas in need of change. If at least the majority of these issues are addressed and resolved in the near future, then this will definitely result in wider adoption of the technology and an overall improvement of health services and outcomes for the population at large.

7.4 CASE STUDIES

As mHealth technology continues to grow and impact people's lives, some targeted applications have also been deployed with positive results, especially in developing countries where access to healthcare is often limited due to several reasons. In this section we present a few of such case studies or use cases briefly.

7.4.1 Case Studies: Viamo and mHealth Apps

Viamo[3] is a global social enterprise that leverages the power of mobile technology to bring positive changes in individuals and organizations. It particularly specializes in using the power of digital technology in countries and regions that do not have the infrastructure to allow access to good healthcare and information related to healthcare. This has led to significant improvements in patient-provider communication and relationships and enhanced medical and health-related knowledge for patients, thus creating overall better health outcomes. Details about all these case studies may be obtained from [5]. All of these are noteworthy efforts and have contributed significantly to enhancing healthcare delivery and outcomes in developing countries around the globe. Not only that, but such efforts also show the potential opportunities for other technology-based companies to undertake similar projects and even develop new and more innovative healthcare solutions in order to make healthcare accessible and beneficial to more and more individuals.

7.4.1.1 Patient Case Management

Viamo has helped in integrating IVR (interactive voice response) services with case management platforms to facilitate the communication and interaction between patients and healthcare workers via mobile phones, thus improving the quality and delivery of care. This has been implemented in Zambia for male circumcision clients and in Senegal for an exchange of messages between the patients and healthcare workers regarding side effects (of drugs or surgeries) tracking and reminders about upcoming appointments.

7.4.1.2 Disease Prevention

IVRs have been employed in countries like Sierra Leone via an integration of Viamo with their local healthcare platforms to promote Ebola vaccination campaigns, encourage patients to adhere to treatment regimens and follow healthy practices, and enable healthcare workers to remotely monitor patients and communicate with them as needed. The data were also analyzed in real-time to provide a map of disease outbreak and determine demographic trends that facilitated appropriate infectious disease management and mitigation measures.

7.4.1.3 Diagnostics

In Ghana and the Democratic Republic of the Congo (DRC), Viamo has helped UNICEF with using IVR services for the early detection of life-threatening diseases, like malaria and yellow fever, by providing diagnostic advice, self-diagnostic services, and treatment options. These types of free live and on-demand tailored health services have reached even people who previously had no access to healthcare.

7.4.1.4 Data Management

Since 2011, Viamo has helped Madagascar's Ministry of Health to strengthen its health systems by collecting real-time data on disease outbreaks and stock monitoring for vital drugs (so that they do not run out in case of an outbreak). Such data are submitted regularly via mobile devices by health workers that are immediately available for tracking by their health system.

7.4.1.5 Surveillance and Monitoring

Viamo has helped the country of Afghanistan to eradicate polio, along with UNICEF, via their IVR services to continuously monitor patients remotely and track the number of monthly vaccinations. This has greatly helped healthcare workers to understand high-risk populations for such diseases, provide accurate information to patients in a timely manner, and arrange for suitable and adequate care by freeing up other resources.

7.4.1.6 Audio Job Aids

Viamo is helping to train community healthcare workers in Bihar, India, about life-saving health behaviors via audio-based courses delivered through their IVR services. The workers are able to access these trainings at any time from their mobile phones and can complete the trainings at their own pace. This is a great initiative and helps overcome barriers by fulfilling real-time training needs assessments and ongoing evaluations of care providers' knowledge requisite knowledge, skills, and competencies in the relevant areas.

7.4.2 Case Study: Physical Fitness Trackers

Just as with mHealth apps, there have been several case studies to explore the positive impacts of physical or wearable fitness tracking devices on different aspects of one's health, such as physical activity, sleep, chronic pain management, and mental health. We include brief details of a couple of these below, but more details can be found from the individual references. For more case studies with Fitbit trackers, the reader is referred to the Fitbit health solutions website [6].

7.4.2.1 Mental Health, Sleep, and Physical Activity

Mental health issues like depression are common in stressful work environments, which was exacerbated by the COVID-19 pandemic beginning in March of 2020. Given the difficulty in getting access to suitable mental healthcare services in a timely fashion, depression rates are hard to reduce. Hence alternative methods to address these issues via mHealth technology are needed. [7] conducted a micro-randomized trial over a six-month period involving 1,565 subjects who were in the medical profession. These participants were provided with a Fitbit Charge 2 device, and the mobile app was downloaded to their phones. Every week, these subjects were assigned to different groups that received different types of push notifications related to a particular category, such as mood, activity, sleep, or no notifications ('control' group). The subjects were also asked to log their daily mood valence, sleep, and step counts. The purpose of the study was to investigate the effects of the notification messages from the tracker as interventions to improve mental and overall health via statistical moderation analysis.

The results indicated that the notifications had a better impact on mood, sleep, and physical activity when the subjects had a 'low' week before in

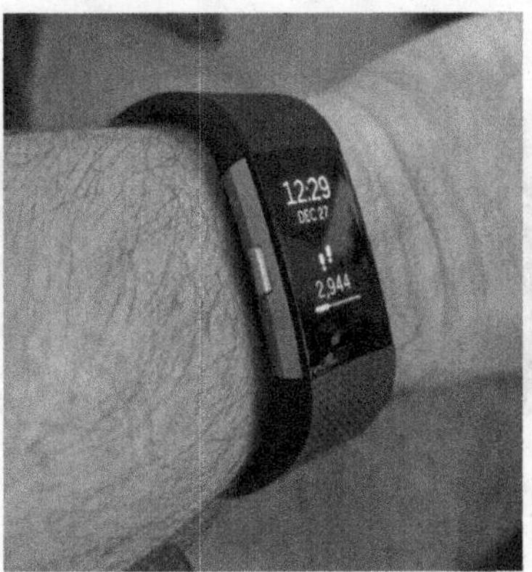

FIGURE 7.3 Fitbit charge 2 device (License: CC.)

terms of mood, sleep, and step counts respectively. Thus, the interventions provided by the fitness tracker proved to be beneficial in improving both health and mental health conditions to a considerable extent. The authors further concluded from their analysis that timing such interventions to match a person's current state may be the key to maximizing the efficacy of such interventions.

7.4.2.2 Chronic Pain

Wearable fitness trackers have been found to help with self-health and wellness management. Hence it is believed that they can help people manage chronic conditions such as musculoskeletal pain. Older adults and especially those belonging to minority groups, who are more vulnerable to such chronic conditions, face obstacles to using fitness trackers. [8] conducted a research case study among 51 African American adult males aged between 60 and 85 years and living in an economically disadvantaged community who suffered from chronic musculoskeletal pain. A randomized control trial was designed with 28 people in an 'intervention' group who were provided with a Fitbit Zip tracker and 23 assigned to the 'control' group (no tracker was provided). The purpose of the study was to evaluate whether the intervention in the form of a wearable device was associated with improvements in pain and walking frequency. The intervention group participants were required to report their daily step counts recorded by the Fitbit device via text messages, automated phone calls, and syncing with the associated Fitbit mobile app. The study duration was six weeks.

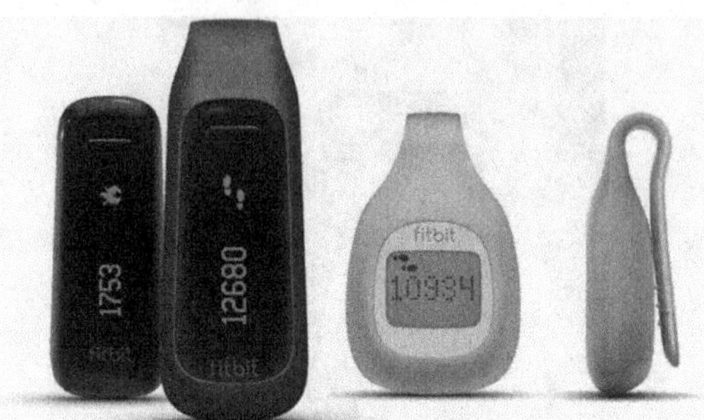

FIGURE 7.4 Fitbit zip device (License: CC.)

The results found that more than 90% of the subjects found the wearable Fitbit device easy to use, although some reported technical issues with the device or with the app for reporting the steps. Final findings showed that while 75% of the intervention group members said that the Fitbit motivated them to walk more, no significant improvement was observed in terms of pain interference. Despite these results, this case study established the promising fact that it is feasible to use physical fitness tracking devices for chronic pain self-care among the vulnerable older population with appropriate needs-based support. In fact, some research studies have shown the potential of fitness trackers like pedometers in managing other chronic health conditions, such as diabetes, hypertension, arthritis, and cardiovascular diseases [9].

7.5 THE ROAD AHEAD: NEW OPPORTUNITIES AND AREAS OF GROWTH

According to a World Health Organization (WHO) report from 2019 [10], higher-income countries show more mHealth activity than do lower-income countries. Countries in Europe are currently the most active and those in the Africa the least active. mHealth is most easily incorporated into processes and services that historically use voice communication through conventional telephone networks. Since then, the advanced functionalities of mobile phones, such as text messaging, Bluetooth, and others, have been used to design and develop more sophisticated mHealth applications. However, lower-income countries often do not have reliable internet connectivity and wireless technology everywhere, especially in remote areas, and a large subset of the population does not own a smartphone. Thus, there is an acute need to expand internet, wireless, and mobile technology in such countries where citizens also have restricted access to healthcare owing to lack of infrastructure and resources so that the use of mHealth services can be increased significantly. As seen with the Viamo case studies, there are organizations that are spearheading such efforts. More organizations can get involved in similar and newer initiatives, which have the potential to cause a paradigm shift in how healthcare is used and delivered across the globe.

Strategically planned and rigorous evaluation techniques and large-scale research studies are critical in educating the public about the benefits of mHealth; hence the strategic planning and development of such activities are needed to enhance the impact of mHealth and lead to effective policy making. The latter will become even more important as the field of mHealth develops and matures, the key component being related to data security and privacy. There are legitimate concerns about the security of information collected and stored by mHealth technologies, and any breaches can put the personal information of the users of the technology at serious risk. Policy makers and program managers thus need to be made aware of such security issues in the mHealth domain so that appropriate policies and strategies can be developed and implemented. Policies will definitely prove to be vital to efforts in harmonizing eHealth and mHealth initiatives and directions in the short- and long-term [10].

In conclusion, many innovations are still possible in the mHealth technology world, and the future is extremely bright and ripe with opportunities for both researchers and technology developers to bring about revolutionary changes in how healthcare is delivered today in the United States and across the globe. This kind of transformation will be driven primarily by the continual explosive growth of technology, and in particular, the advances in mobile technology and applications along with Internet of Things (IoT) devices, that can facilitate the integration of mobile health with existing health services in a very convenient way. As with any technology, this will be possible with the required effort on part of the mHealth technology companies to understand the underlying issues and concerns and address them adequately.

NOTES

1 www.ralphlauren.com/rlmag/polotech-cardio.html?ab=en_US_rlmag_polotech-strength_L1

2 www.sensoriafitness.com/smartsocks/

3 https://viamo.io/about-viamo/

REFERENCES

1. Grandview Research (2021). mHealth Market Size, Share & Trends Analysis Report by Component (mHealth Apps, Wearables), by Services (Diagnosis, Monitoring), By Participants (Mobile Operators, Content Players), and Segment Forecasts. Link: www.grandviewresearch.com/industry-analysis/mhealth-market, published in February 2021. Retrieved on September 27, 2021.
2. Global Market Insights Report (2021). Link: www.gminsights.com/industry-analysis/mhealth-market, published in April 2021. Retrieved on September 27, 2021.
3. Hunt, R. (2021). 13 Best Smart Clothing for Performance and Health (2021 Update). *The VOU*. Link: https://thevou.com/fashion/smart-clothing/, published on February 12, 2021. Retrieved on September 28, 2021.
4. Gokey, M., Lord, S. (2021). The best smart jewelry in 2021, from necklaces to rings and watches, *Business Insider*. Link: www.businessinsider.com/best-smart-jewelry, published on March 31, 2021. Retrieved on September 28, 2021.
5. Viamo case studies. Link: https://viamo.io/case-studies/, retrieved on October 9, 2021.
6 Fitbit Health Solutions. Link: https://healthsolutions.fitbit.com/research-library/, retrieved on October 11, 2021.
7. NeCamp, T., Sen, S., Frank, E., Walton, M.A., Ionides, E.L., Fang, Y., Tewari, A., Wu, Z. (2020). Assessing Real-Time Moderation for Developing Adaptive Mobile Health Interventions for Medical Interns: Micro-Randomized Trial, *Journal of Medical Internet Research*, 22(3): e15033. DOI: 10.2196/15033
8. Janevic, M., Murphy, S., Shute, V., Piette, J. (2019). Acceptability and effects of using wearable activity trackers for chronic pain management among older African American adults, *The Journal of Pain*, 20(4) Supplement, pp: S67–68.
9. Gierisch, J.G., Goode, A.P., Allen, K.D., Batch, B.C., Shaw, R.J. (2015). The Impact of Pedometers on Chronic Conditions – A Review of Reviews, *White paper, Department of Veterans Affairs*, Durham, NC.
10. World Health Organization. mHealth: New horizons for health through mobile technologies. Available online, link: www.who.int/goe/publications/goe_mhealth_web.pdf. Retrieved on October 4, 2021.

Index

Note: Page numbers in *italic* denote figures and in **bold** denote tables.

Printed in the United States
by Baker & Taylor Publisher Services

Printed in the United States
by Baker & Taylor Publisher Services